T0143291

Developing a Narrative Approach to Healthcare Research

Developing a Narrative Approach to Healthcare Research

VIV MARTIN

PhD

Foreword by

Karen Forbes

Radcliffe Publishing

Oxford • New York

Radcliffe Publishing Ltd
18 Marcham Road
Abingdon
Oxon OX14 1AA
United Kingdom

www.radcliffepublishing.com
Electronic catalogue and worldwide online ordering facility.

© 2011 Viv Martin

Viv Martin has asserted her right under the Copyright, Designs and Patents Act 1998 to be identified as the author of this work.

All rights reserved. No part of this publication may be reproduced, stored in a retrieval system or transmitted, in any form or by any means, electronic, mechanical, photocopying, recording or otherwise, without the prior permission of the copyright owner.

British Library Cataloguing in Publication Data

A catalogue record for this book is available from the British Library.

ISBN-13: 978 184619 400 9

The paper used for the text pages of this book is FSC certified. FSC (The Forest Stewardship Council) is an international network to promote responsible management of the world's forests.

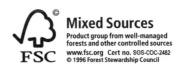

Mixed Sources
Product group from well-managed forests and other controlled sources
www.fsc.org Cert no. SGS-COC-2482
© 1996 Forest Stewardship Council

Typeset by KnowledgeWorks Global Ltd, Chennai, India
Printed and bound by TJI Digital, Padstow, Cornwall, UK

Contents

Foreword

I first met Viv Martin while sitting in a narrative workshop in the Graduate School of Education at the University of Bristol. My admiration for her grew as I learnt of her story and was, in small ways, involved in the unfolding of the journey that brings her to the publication of this book—and me to the honour of being asked to write the foreword for it. I am a consultant in palliative medicine involved in medical education and interested in narrative both as a way of hearing my students' stories and as a tool to explore their experiences of learning to look after people who are very ill and dying. I have cared for many people during their journeys through illness. Viv has been there; she is a remarkable lady.

Many, faced with life-threatening illness, surgery that could kill or severely disable, and the ongoing spectre of further problems, would awaken each morning, pinch themselves and be glad merely to be alive. Not Viv. Once she could write, having had to learn to do so with her non-dominant hand, she wrote—fascinated by the way in which writing and storytelling helped her to understand the person she had been before her surgery, the process she had been through and the person that thinking about, telling and writing her story had helped her to become. She published her first book, *Out of my Head*, an account of her journey through neurosurgery and her meaning-making during that journey in 1997. Her realisation of the importance of narrative and story in finding her new place in the world led her to explore whether narrative and story had been as pivotal for others. The result was her doctoral thesis and now this book.

In this book, Viv gathers together the stories of four very different people who have faced disability, illness and surgery: Pat, an experienced dialysis nurse facing kidney failure; Jan, facing the spectre of ever more surgery for congenital hip problems; Jim, experiencing sudden, unexpected heart disease and surgery; and Yasmin, undergoing the roller coaster of remissions and exacerbations of severe inflammatory bowel disease. But this book is not just about telling stories, it is also a celebration of the individuals telling those stories and of storytelling: of the power of stories to shape and heal lives, to make and regain identity and to assert the uniqueness and personhood of the story teller. Viv then goes on to tell and examine the story of her research process, the ethics of asking people to tell their stories and of presenting them to others, the responsibility of representation and the implications of it, weaving throughout rich diverse narrative literature. Her reason for doing so is clear:

> A nurse who read one of my contributors' stories commented, "This should be read by the nurses on the ward – they tend to forget that this is a person with a life." When I asked my contributors what message they particularly wanted to get across, everyone indicated the importance of being recognised as a person.

She suggests:

> The relational dimension of narrative encompasses both our singularity and our shared humanity. I would add that if we learn to *tend* our own stories, and to acknowledge our own vulnerabilities, then we are more likely to *attend to* and bear witness to the stories of others.

Viv's contributors wanted to be recognised as people; she has certainly recognised them as such, tending and attending to their stories with great care; they are nurtured and shaped to powerful effect. But for whom? Who should read this book? Anyone interested in narrative as method, but I hope that healthcare professionals will also read it. Medical students, for instance, become increasingly 'professionalised' during their training. They learn to adopt professional distance so that they do not become enmeshed in—and disabled by—the emotional impact of the situations they encounter. Some are so good at this they lose sight of the person behind the diagnosis. Jim's story, for instance, is 'ordinary': a heart attack, coronary artery bypass grafting ... it happens every day to countless people. But this book shows us the man behind the diagnosis, the impact of what has happened to him on his identity, on him as a unique individual. Viv does this so well; I find some of her deft, small touches—the green doors, the red shoes—unbelievably moving.

I will recommend this book to my students; I hope other healthcare professionals will do the same and that some, like me, will go on to explore how narrative and story can be harnessed to both explore experience and to teach within healthcare.

Karen Forbes
Consultant and Macmillan Professorial Teaching Fellow in Palliative Medicine
University Hospitals Bristol NHS Foundation Trust and University of Bristol

Preface

INTRODUCTION

Stories form the basis of this book. At its heart are the illness stories told to me in narrative research conversations with Pat, Ian, Jim and Yasmin, as well as an account of my own illness; these were the basis for a narrative inquiry into the experience of illness and its impact on the identities of five people.

Stories have long had their place in medicine—traditionally in the form of the 'case study', a form of professional narrative that focuses on a single 'case'. If narrative is a *re*-presentation of events over time told to a particular audience, then the 'case' fulfils these criteria: it involves the selection and shaping of a sequence of relevant events and the presentation of these events to a prospective audience. As a representation and medical interpretation of facts and events, the case report will usually be written in the third person to remove any suggestion of subjectivity or expression of emotion. However, those same events told by a patient to a friend will be conveyed from a different perspective to a different audience; the portrayal of events will be subjective and convey feelings, values and interpretations that give meaning to the events within a particular life in relation to a personal or social context. Similarly, a doctor's account of her/his day at work as told to a partner will express experiential knowledge from a particular personal perspective in a particular relational context.

What researchers bring to their task, in terms of both personal and professional knowledge, often connects with their own life stories, and my interest in this research originated in my own experience of illness. With a professional background in teaching and counselling, and following major disruption to my life through serious illness and neurosurgery, I ventured into autobiographical writing. Together with an emerging interest in narrative ideas and practices, this led me to undertake a PhD at the University of Bristol. My doctorate was a narrative inquiry in which I worked with four people who had experienced major health problems; I examined the impact of health difficulties on their lives and identities. In a sense, this book is an account of that research; it is an empirically based text that is both a collection of illness stories and a reflection on the process of collecting those stories.

The book attempts to show that both patient stories and practitioner stories are significant within healthcare settings. Patient stories have the capacity to touch the hearts and minds of healthcare professionals; by illustrating and giving insight into illness experience, they contribute 'narrative' knowledge which can enhance the practice of ethical and effective healthcare.[1] Within medical education, the pioneering work of practitioner educators such as Rita Charon[2] has demonstrated the impact that training in narrative approaches can make on the practice of healthcare workers. Indeed, Charon reports that ongoing research into the outcomes of narrative reflective writing (which she terms 'Parallel Charts') has shown that practitioners were 'more effective in conducting medical interviews, performing medical procedures, and developing therapeutic alliances with patients' (p. 174). Clandinin and Cave[3] have developed Charon's idea of the 'Parallel Chart' and also note the beneficial impact on clinical skills. Narrative reflective writing has been shown to enhance sensitive and critical examination of practice, and thus to contribute to the personal and professional development of healthcare practitioners.[4,5,6,7,8] Whether we are positioned as practitioners or as patients (or both), we all have stories to tell, and this book explores the way those stories are intimately bound up with identity construction in both personal and professional domains.

NARRATIVE

The concept of narrative has gained an increasingly high profile in recent years within the health and social sciences. Narrative approaches to human knowledge rest principally on the idea that one of the fundamental ways in which we organise and make sense of our lives, the lives of others and the world in which we live is through telling stories. Stories capture individual, collective and social ways of being-in-the-world, and, as has been claimed across many disciplines, are central to our ways of making meaning. As John McLeod[9] writes in his introduction to *Narrative and Psychotherapy*, 'stories represent the basic means by which people organise and communicate the meaning of events and experiences' (p. x). We tell stories about ourselves and others as part of our daily lives. Stories appear in a range of cultural settings and genres: we read autobiographies, fictional novels, poetry, fairy tales; we watch television soaps, theatrical or cinematic dramas, films of everyday life as well as epic adventure, political intrigue, and tales of fantasy. To some extent, the terms 'narrative' and 'story' are used interchangeably; however, McLeod,[10] writing in the field of psychotherapy, distinguishes 'story' as an 'account of a specific event' from 'narrative' as a 'story-based account of happenings' that contains 'other forms of communication in addition to stories' (p. 31). While 'story' is a word in everyday use, 'narrative' is a term drawn from literary studies, which is used in academic discourse and has also found its way into popular discourse. We may encounter it across a range of media, political and social contexts. In cultural forms such as drama, film, dance, poetry or novels, 'narrative' is used to indicate a line of causal or thematic progression.

Psychologist Jerome Bruner[11] has made the distinction between a paradigmatic approach to knowledge and a narrative approach; both provide necessary means for us to make sense of the world. He regards these modes of thought as providing distinctive and different ways of organising experience and constructing reality. While the paradigmatic mode of thinking represents knowledge in conceptual and propositional terms, narrative knowing focuses on the particulars of lived experience in the form of stories and pays attention to the temporal unfolding of human lives, as well as their personal, social and cultural meanings. Furthermore, he regards narrative, not just as a way in which we make meaning of our lives, but also as fundamental to the construction of selfhood—a view substantiated, as we shall see, across the human sciences.[12,13] (*See* Chapter Eight for further discussion.) The stories we tell are influenced by cultural models of selfhood but also have an influence on the selves we construct; the stories that follow in chapters One to Five and the issues they highlight (Chapters Six and Seven) illustrate something of this interplay between personal agency and implicit cultural models of identity.

NARRATIVE INQUIRY

The social sciences have developed out of the natural sciences where questions of what constitutes valid research are based on a view of knowledge informed by paradigmatic thinking and the values of objectivity, impartiality and generalisability. The status and authority of a scientific approach to knowledge has therefore influenced views of what constitutes 'proper' research in the social sciences. Narrative approaches to research, on the other hand, contribute subjectivity, partiality and particularity as complementary knowledge. Criteria for evaluating narrative research are therefore associated with knowledge claims that value their capacity to represent personal, everyday, experiential and culturally situated knowledge that will resonate with others and perhaps shed light on human experience, thereby influencing attitudes, transforming practice and having personal, social and political impact. I will discuss questions of validity and evaluation more fully in Part Three of this book.

Narrative inquiry encompasses a broad, diverse range of qualitative approaches to social research. There is wide variation in how researchers conceptualise 'narrative' as a means and method for exploring, representing and understanding human experience; narrative can refer to a range of theoretical orientations and methodologies as well as topics of study. How we view the world, our view of what constitutes knowledge, and what it means to be human will inform the way we position ourselves as narrative researchers and the methodologies through which we approach our field of interest.

NARRATIVE AND HEALTHCARE

The experience of sickness has a tremendous impact on all of us. It affects individuals, families, communities and society; illness does not occur in a vacuum, but in everyday experiences that are situated within social contexts. It influences interactions within a person's family, work and community environments; it not only changes the structure of life stories, it has an impact on selfhood and raises existential questions about meaning, purpose and identity. Becoming a 'patient' highlights the relationship between knowledge and power; it alerts us to issues of difference, inclusion and social marginalisation. The experience of illness therefore has implications for any of us wherever and however we are positioned within society.

The view within psychology and the social sciences that people are active social beings who structure their personal and cultural realities through narrative and storytelling has been recognised within medicine, where writers such as Charon,[14] Brody,[15] Kleinman[16] and Mishler[17] have made major contributions that have highlighted the importance of narrative in clinical practice and education. Research in health and illness is at the interface of science and life, and narrative approaches have gained increasing recognition as methods which can offer, as neurologist Oliver Sacks expresses it, 'a crucial counterbalance to the medical, the impersonal, scientific description of us as cases' (personal communication). Personal stories, which provide multi-faceted, detailed pictures of individual illness experience, can contribute knowledge that complements medical accounts and case notes, and thereby illuminate and inform healthcare practice.

In their introduction to *Narrative Research in Health and Illness*, Hurwitz *et al.*[18] suggest that narrative-based approaches have developed in response to a prevailing scientific and rationalist view of health and illness where they have acted as a means of mediating between the specialist literature on narrative in disciplines such as anthropology, philosophy and literary studies. They highlight the way that 'Narrative ... expresses the uniqueness of each person and addresses the listener, not as a professional, but as a fellow human being' (p. 1). This intersubjective dimension of narrative has long been recognised by those such as Charon,[19] Kleinman[20] and Frank,[21] who emphasise the importance of engaging with stories as an interpersonal and ethical act. Rita Charon, in particular, has developed a narrative approach to clinical practice which is informed by literary insight, involves a commitment to listening to stories and a willingness to relate as a fellow human being.

The influence of the humanities and arts upon research in health and illness has enabled the development of approaches which represent personal, affective and relational aspects of experience, rather than the objective, evidence-based discourse of the clinical case. Collaborative, participatory approaches to research and the development of arts-based methodologies have opened up possibilities for imaginative exploration of experience which might draw on (for example) poetry, art, drama or the techniques of the novel for representing subjectivities. Such approaches to narrative inquiry have contributed to the development of ethical and aesthetic research *with* participants, in contrast to more traditional models of research *on* subjects.

QUESTIONS OF SELFHOOD AND IDENTITY

In his book *Into the Silent Land*, neuropsychologist Paul Broks[22] touches on many issues that relate to embodiment and sense of self, and he highlights the fundamental role of narrative as a means of making sense of life. Broks tells compelling tales of his encounters and personal engagements with his patients, and he combines personal reflections on his professional practice with the stories of people whose lives are disrupted by the contingency and chaos of neurological injury or illness. As well as describing the material substance and physiology of the brain and exploring its networks and capacities, Broks raises questions on the nature of selfhood. In an era when neuroscience is developing the technology to reveal the minute details of the neurobiological basis of the mind, Broks observes:

> What became clear was that the brain could not be fully understood if you treated it as an isolated object. I had underestimated how tightly our brain's functions are tied to the rest of our body, and at the same time, how deeply they are embedded in the wider physical and social landscape. No brain is an island. (p. 49)

I find personal resonance in many of the stories in his book; they evoke my own experience of illness and reawaken my curiosity and fascination with the mysteries of consciousness. Who are the selves we believe ourselves to be? And what happens to those selves when we are anaesthetised? How do we preserve some sense of identity when we are inert bodies on an operating table? How do we find, maintain, create or recreate a sense of self in the face of serious health problems or life-threatening illness? What is the relationship between our personal embodiment and the social and cultural context in which we live? And what is the role of narrative in this?

But Broks raises not only questions of identity and consciousness; his metaphor of the 'silent land' reminds me of illness stories that go untold. This may be for many reasons; perhaps they seem paradoxical or contradictory; or perhaps dominant discourses decree which stories are acceptable or unacceptable. Perhaps such stories are too painful to tell or to hear. Or perhaps there is simply too much to tell; Pat, who recounts her experience of renal failure in Chapter Two, expresses this clearly: 'As I'm talking to you, I'm reliving some of it in my head. I'm telling you bits of it, but in my mind I can see the whole scenario playing out … and the emotions. I'm telling you part of it, but in my mind the rest of it is happening.'

STRUCTURE OF THE BOOK

Personal stories constitute the first section of the book from Chapters One to Five. I introduce the stories from Pat, Jan, Jim and Yasmin with an autoethnographic account of my own illness story and identity transformations, in which I reflect on my positioning in relation to this research project; here I reflect on the relationship between my counselling background, the impact of illness on my life and identity, and the way in which these informed my research relationships and the development of my methodology.

In Part Two, I widen my interpretive gaze to look across all five stories and focus on the dimensions of illness experience which the narratives highlight. In Chapter Six, I examine imagery in the stories: figurative language encountered or used in the form of metaphor and simile. In Chapter Seven, I focus on particular issues raised by the storytellers. I do not claim an absolute definitive exploration of issues nor thematic analysis of the stories; rather, I highlight themes that seem to me to be pertinent; I acknowledge that my perception of these dimensions of illness experience is partial and do not foreclose on interpretations which readers may bring to the stories in this book.

In Part Three, I examine the concepts that underpin narrative approaches to research and focus particularly on the evolution of the relational approach to narrative inquiry that developed out of my experience as a counsellor, patient and writer. I make links between narrative ideas and practices and the implications of these for healthcare education, practice and research. Chapters Eight to Ten focus on methodological considerations: in Chapter Eight, I offer a rationale and justification for employing a narrative approach to researching the impact of illness on identity and life course, and examine the concepts on which this research is based. Chapter Nine addresses questions of research design and method, and how these are interwoven with issues of ethics, accountability and questions of validity: I examine the nature of my relationships with those who contributed their stories, and the values on which my approach to narrative inquiry is based. I describe the development of my particular approach to narrative inquiry and outline the broad framework for meetings with participants. I discuss questions of ethics and accountability before going on to consider how we might evaluate this kind of research. Chapter Ten focuses on questions of representation, and how I moved between research conversations, transcriptions and the *re*-presentations in Parts One and Two. Supplementary material relating to these chapters is available online at: www.radcliffepublishing.com/devnarrativehcres/

The two final chapters focus on the relevance of this project for medical education and practice, and for research. In Chapter Eleven, I consider the implications of these stories for healthcare practice. In Chapter Twelve, I draw the book to a close with some reflections on methodological issues and on my personal learning over the course of this project.

AN INVITATION

Heather Leach,[23] in a challenge to the 'relentless forward linearity of narrative', suggests that 'experience may be outside narrative … what surrounds, what threatens the path of the life, is fearful, chaotic, confusing' (p. 18). In the stories that follow, I have tried to convey something of the chaos of experience and to represent a sense of the dialogic and relational nature of the storytelling process; I invite the reader to engage with the stories and to enter into relation with them—and, in Arthur Frank's words,[24] to 'listen *with*' the storytellers. I hope that the stories, together with the issues and concerns they raise, may contribute knowledge which—though situated, personal and partial—is also collective and potentially transformative of healthcare practice: knowledge that has the potential to enrich and inform professional and social attitudes and policy.

I believe the tales told by Oliver Sacks[25,26,27] and Irvin Yalom[28] 'work' because they are compelling stories, beautifully told, which invite us into the lives of others: tales which arouse our curiosities but above all engage our empathy and imagination. Stories are relational; they invite affective engagement and interaction. In my representations of the stories of Pat, Jan, Jim and Yasmin, I set out to encompass both the personal and socio-cultural dimensions of illness and identity construction. My aim was to create compelling, resonant texts which communicated the immediacy and particularities of each personal narrative as well as a sense of my own positioning, the relational nature of our research conversations, and the ways in which the stories were shaped through dialogue and co-construction. Above all, I have tried to honour and do justice to their experiences and the stories they have entrusted to me. This introduction is an invitation to the reader to engage with these stories; they tell of hope and despair, of vitality and mortality, of vulnerability and strength, of meaning-making and of the absence of meaning, of wounds that can heal and those that can never heal.

A NOTE ABOUT LANGUAGE AND TERMINOLOGY

I use more than one term for the people who took part in this research project. We are variously co-researcher/participant/co-participant/interviewee/storyteller[29]/contributor.[30] While each of these terms signify practices and positioning, I blur them deliberately for stylistic reasons and also in order to reflect my awareness of language as an arena of struggle where meanings are claimed, selves are positioned and understandings are mediated through discourses considered appropriate to particular fields or domains of knowledge. I have therefore decided to use the terms interchangeably; I am clearly in the role of researcher but also a participant and storyteller alongside Jan, Jim, Pat and Yasmin. Bridges[31] experienced similar dilemmas over how to refer to the people involved in her project and decided to use the term 'contributors', since 'this reflects the active nature of their input and acknowledges my inevitable ownership of the project' (p. 6). I therefore gratefully borrow the word 'contributor'.

NARRATIVE/STORY/STORIES

To some extent, I use narrative and story interchangeably in this book; I use 'narrative' as a wider, more generic and academic term, and 'story' as a more accessible term to refer to a personal account of events over time. I use 'stories' when I am referring to all five stories in the study. I also use it when I am referring to the interwoven stories of one person. Thus a 'story' may comprise separate stories that are linked together in an overarching narrative.

REFERENCES

1. Bleakley A, Marshall R, Bromer R. Toward an aesthetic medicine: developing a core medical humanities undergraduate curriculum. *J Med Humanit.* 2006; **27**: 197–213.
2. Charon R. *Narrative Medicine: honoring the stories of illness.* Oxford: Oxford University Press; 2006.
3. Clandinin DJ, Cave MT. Creating pedagogical spaces for developing doctor professional identity. *Med Educ.* 2008; **42**: 765–70.
4. Charon, op cit.
5. Clandinin, Cave, op cit.
6. Clandinin DJ, Cave MT. Storytelling in Medicine. Available at: www.expressnews.ualberta.ca/article.cfm?id=8246.
7. Bolton G. *Reflective Practice Writing and Professional Development.* London: Sage; 2005.
8. Feest K, Forbes K. *Today's Students, Tomorrow's Doctors.* Oxford: Radcliffe; 2007.
9. McLeod J. *Narrative and Psychotherapy.* London: Sage; 1997.
10. Ibid.
11. Bruner J. *Actual Minds, Possible Worlds.* Cambridge, MA: Harvard University Press; 1986.
12. Bruner J. *Acts of Meaning.* Cambridge, MA: Harvard University Press; 1990.
13. Bruner J. *Making Stories: law, literature, life.* New York, NY: Farrar, Straus and Giroux; 2002.
14. Charon, op cit.
15. Brody H. *Stories of Sickness.* New Haven, CT: Yale University Press; 1987.
16 Kleinman A. *The Illness Narratives: suffering, healing and the human condition.* New York, NY: Basic Books; 1988.
17. Mishler EG. *The Discourse of Medicine: dialectics of medical interviews.* Norwood, NJ: Ablex Publishing Corp; 1984.
18. Hurwitz B, Greenhalgh T, Skultans V, editors. *Narrative Research in Health and Illness.* London: BMJ Books; 2004.
19 Charon, op cit.
20. Kleinman, op cit.
21. Frank A. *The Wounded Storyteller: body, illness and ethics.* Chicago, IL: University of Chicago Press; 1995.
22. Broks P. *Into the Silent Land: travels in neuropsychology.* London: Atlantic Books; 2004.
23. Leach H. Crossing the line: stories on mapping the maze. *Times Higher Education Supplement.* 2004 Nov. 5; 18–19.
24. Frank, op cit.
25. Sacks O. *Awakenings.* London: Gerald Duckworth and Co; 1973.
26. Sacks O. *The Man Who Mistook His Wife for a Hat.* London: Picador; 1985.
27. Sacks O. *An Anthropologist on Mars.* London: Picador; 1995.
28. Yalom I. *Love's Executioner and Other Tales of Psychotherapy.* Harmondsworth: Penguin; 1989.

29. Etherington K. *Trauma, Drug Misuse and Transforming Identities.* London: Jessica Kingsley; 2008.
30. Bridges N. *Maintaining Ethical Counselling Despite Contrary Demands: a narrative inquiry.* PhD thesis. University of Bristol; 2007.
31. Ibid.

About the author

Viv Martin has a professional background in teaching and counselling. She has taught in primary, secondary, adult, and higher education in the United Kingdom and Zambia. Following serious illness in 1994, she published a book, *Out of my Head*, and journal articles. She worked as a counsellor in bereavement care and higher education before undertaking a PhD at the University of Bristol. Her doctoral research was a narrative inquiry into the impact of illness and surgery on identity and life stories. Her teaching and research interests include narrative inquiry and identity formation in health and illness. She intends to develop future narrative research with healthcare professionals who have personal experience of health problems.

Acknowledgements

This book has been the work of many people; while it carries my name, it also carries the voices of those whose companionship, love, conversations, thoughts and ideas have sustained me over many years.

I am indebted to:

Pat, Jan, Jim and Yasmin for their generosity in taking part in my doctoral research; I have been moved and honoured to work with them, and I thank them for entrusting me with their stories. I hope that I have done justice to their experiences.

Kim Etherington, who was just the most amazing PhD supervisor anyone could wish for. Kim has supported me throughout this research project and beyond; I deeply appreciate her affirmation, wisdom and encouragement as well as her perceptive and constructive comments. Together with her humanity, warmth, generosity of spirit and great hugs, Kim's wonderfully incisive and insightful intellect as well as her gentle and intuitive guidance have played a major role in my becomings and transformations. An abiding and precious memory of spending time with Kim is sharing a pot of tea and drinking from china teacups in a Russian tearoom in the middle of Chicago before setting off for the International Congress of Qualitative Inquiry (ICQI) at the University of Illinois.

Laurinda Brown, who was an invaluable part of my PhD process. Her presence and companionship, wisdom and compassion have sustained me. Our shared musical history has been the source of much joy and fun, and frequent outbursts of singing.

Tim Bond, who has supported, encouraged and believed in me during my time at the University of Bristol. I am immensely grateful to Tim for his insight and engagement throughout this project. I especially enjoyed our conversations about Levinas and Buber over a glass of red wine at the 'old-fashioned Midwest Cookout' during my first trip to ICQI in 2006. I also appreciate his affection for Durham and my native Northeast.

Jane Speedy for her generosity, humour and sparkle. Jane's big heart and creative, subversive spirit continues to enrich my work. Her drive and inspiration have been fundamental to the Bristol Collaborative Writing Group (BCWG). Jane's pivotal role in this research community and in the Centre for Narrative and Transformative Learning has made them invigorating and hugely enjoyable places to be.

Vieda Skultans for her gentle, welcoming presence at the 2004 BMA Narrative Research conference, and her pertinent and helpful support during my PhD.

Karen Forbes for her companionship along the way and her gentle, insightful support.

Thanks to the members of the BCWG: Dave Bainton, Nell Bridges, Laurinda Brown, Artemi Sakellariadis, Jane Speedy, Dick Tahta, Sheila Trahar, Susan Williams and Sue Wilson for inspiration and 'deep hanging out'.

The QI posse: they have varied over the years but have always been wonderful company; we've enjoyed warmth, good humour, and occasionally been a bit 'up ourselves'. Jonathan Wyatt, Ken Gale and Tim Bond were my first companions on the road to ICQI. And it was through QI that my friendships with Jackie Goode, Cindy Gowan, Tami Spry have blossomed.

Kim's conservatory posse: Nell, Ann Dalzell, Ruth Leitch, Ely Samuel and Donna West for ongoing support and email companionship, and hugs when we meet.

I also thank Jackie Goode, Sue May and Carole Pannell, who have inspired and supported me in making my own doctoral journey.

My dear friends Alison and Sue, who have hung in there with me through thick and thin.

Andrew Sparkes and John McLeod, whose support led me to the University of Bristol.

Milne Anderson, Steve Gabriel and Carl Meyer for their part in my story.

Tony Martin, Josie Martin and Steve Martin for their constancy, love and support before, throughout and beyond this project. They have believed in me when I have not believed in myself.

Rosie Martin for her soft purring presence on my desk while I'm writing.

To Sylvia and Albert Scott, and to Tony, Steve and Josie Martin

PART I

Introduction

Chapters One to Five focus on the five illness stories. Each chapter, however, is not *the* illness story of each person: clearly, none is definitive, complete or unequivocal. The stories don't tell everything—nor indeed *can* they tell everything, for as Winterson expresses it, 'There is no everything. The stories themselves make the meaning. The continuous narrative of existence is a lie. There is no continuous narrative, there are lit-up moments and the rest is dark' (p. 134).

While each of the chapters is relatively self-contained, like all stories, they have spaces: they are partial and incomplete. Each one is selective: one version, selected by each narrator, told from a perspective and represented by me (though in consultation with the storytellers). They hold tangents of intersecting storylines, fragments of other people's stories and touch on untold stories. They draw on culturally available storylines, or oft-told personal stories, as well as others that lie at the boundaries of availability. In Part Two, I bring an alternative perspective to my representation of these stories, which will 'light-up' experience differently.

Winterson, J. *Lighthousekeeping*. London: Fourth Estate; 2004.

CHAPTER 1

An autoethnographic introduction

As I have indicated in the Preface, the origins of this book and the research on which it is based lie in my experience of serious illness and neurosurgery in 1994. It was these events that led me to undertake a PhD researching narratives of illness and its impact on identity construction. Prior to my illness, I had worked as a teacher and as a counsellor; however, my experience of life-threatening illness and disability was to lead me into territory I could not have foreseen. In order to account for, and to make explicit, my positioning in relation to the stories in this book and to the particular narrative methodology I developed, I shall tell my own story. In doing so, I aim to contextualise the relational and intersubjective stance I take throughout the book.

There is a sense in which research, for many of us, has its roots in our auto-biographies and our need to make sense of experience through both prospective and retrospective exploration: an unceasing need for exploration that T.S. Eliot captures in his poem 'Little Gidding'.[1] Indeed, Bochner[2] challenges 'the myth that our research is divorced from our lives, that it has no autobiographical dimension, that what we do academically is not part of how we are working through the story of our own life'. Writers from across the social sciences, from disciplines such as anthropology,[3,4] counselling and psychotherapy,[5,6] education,[7,8] and sociology[9,10,11,12] similarly acknowledge the links between life experience and research interests: the relationship between researcher as embodied, socially embedded, interacting individual, and as inherently value-laden. What I bring to this research project is a perspective that is informed by my life experience, concerns, interests and values.

Autoethnography is an autobiographical genre of writing which situates the personal within its social context by combining inquiry into a cultural phenomenon along with personal experience of that phenomenon and ethnographic reflection on it. In doing so, the embodied self of the researcher is recognised as a significant and inherent part of the research process. It is a genre which blurs disciplinary boundaries and is positioned between ethnography and autobiography. Ellis[13] describes autoethnography as 'research, writing, story, and method that connect the autobiographical and personal to the cultural, social and political' (p. xix). Spry[14] (p. 710) defines autoethnography as 'a self-narrative that critiques the situatedness of self with others in social contexts'. There are a variety of approaches to autoethnography, ranging from those that privilege its autobiographical origins[15,16,17] to those emphasising the critical ethnographic study of self within culture (*see* Etherington,[18] Sparkes,[19] Speedy,[20] Spry[21]). This book is broadly autoethnographic in that it is an exploration of a particular social community. I use 'community' here in the sense of the Latin *communitas*, which refers to a grouping based on shared humanity and commonality of experience; in this case, those who have experienced serious illness and surgery. Since it is a community to which I also belong, there is an autobiographical dimension to my interest.

According to McLeod,[22] the key approach to ethnographic research is 'participant observation' in which the researcher spends time 'in the field', immersed in the culture of a particular 'community'. He notes that it is an approach that 'highlights the *differences* between researcher and researched' and that 'this emphasis on difference and cultural distinctiveness raises the question of how far it is possible for someone to understand the experience of others' (p. 65). There is clearly a fundamental question here about the nature of lived experience and the extent to which any of us can fully know and understand the subjectivities of another person. Questions about uniqueness and difference, empathy and identification will be addressed more fully later in this book, but for the present, I want to suggest that my 'insider knowledge' of serious illness gives me some access to and understanding of the illness community, which bridges something of the difference between researcher and researched and recognises our shared humanity; I am positioned as co-participant as well as researcher and belong to the community I am researching. Church[23] (p. 3) emphasises the social dimension of the subjective and describes how in her work with 'psychiatric survivors ... the realities of genuine engagement made it virtually impossible not to take up subjectivity'. Likewise, to situate myself solely as counsellor-researcher would be to situate Pat, Jan, Jim and Yasmin as 'other', rather than to acknowledge the place of my own autobiography in this research project and in my relationships with them.

A HEURISTIC JOURNEY

At a gathering in 2003 with my research supervisor, Kim Etherington, and three of her other research students, we were invited to tell our 'research stories'.[24] It was a profound and moving experience; and one that affirmed for me something I have known for a long time, but also that I forget time and time again. It was the most powerful reminder of my deeper knowledge that whatever we experience in life is a stage in the process leading us to where we are and who we are now. We had all taken very different routes, and none of us could have known in advance where those routes were leading. That day, at Kim's house, our particular paths crossed, and in their crossing, reaffirmed for me the validity of each person's path, and reminded me that what we bring to research is fundamentally connected with who we are as persons.

At around the same time, while watching the film *The Matrix*[25] with my daughter, we both noticed the line, 'There is a difference between knowing the path and walking the path'. It would not have occurred to me to venture into research. It was not something I had planned; the path I have taken has been the result of life events and choices that have led me in this direction—not a direction I could possibly have foreseen—but one that makes sense to me retrospectively.

The origins of heuristic research lie in hermeneutics and in Gadamer's notion of the 'horizon of understanding', which refers to our pre-understandings, or assumptions. Hermeneutics involves a dialogic relationship between the researcher and the 'text' or field of inquiry to arrive at a 'fusion of horizons'[26] (p. 290) where the aim is to bridge the gap between the world of the interpreter and the world of the interpreted. As McLeod[27] writes:

> Every act of hermeneutic understanding begins with a pre-understanding which orients the inquirer in relation to the text or topic. One of the tasks of the hermeneutic scholar is to become aware of and reflexively to explicate this pre-understanding in a way that creatively feeds in to the process of understanding itself. (p. 23)

However, Heuristic Inquiry as developed by Moustakas refers to a particular form of phenomenological investigation into human experience. It is an approach that requires the researcher's personal connection to the topic and willingness to engage actively and deeply with it. Moustakas[28] writes, 'The heuristic process is autobiographic, yet with virtually every question that matters personally there is also a social - perhaps universal - significance' (p. 15). He describes the beginnings of heuristic inquiry in terms that are reminiscent of a quest, and writes:

> I begin the heuristic journey with something that has called to me from within my life experiences, and something to which I have associations and fleeting awarenesses but whose nature is largely unknown. In such an odyssey I know little of the territory through which I must travel. (p. 13)

The nature of this journey, then, is that it seeks to illuminate a topic that has personal significance for the researcher and also has wider human/social implications. I am aware of how profoundly and how broadly my personal history influenced my choice of research topic as well as the evolution of the methodology I used; in this chapter, I aim to show how the particular path I have travelled has informed my research interests as well as the underlying philosophy and values which underpin my methodological choices. The research on which this book is based was part of my own quest to understand those 'associations and fleeting awarenesses': a quest which involves looking within, and also reaching outwards in community with others.

WRITING VULNERABLY

Behar[29] observes that 'writing vulnerably' requires us 'to draw deeper connections between one's personal experience and the subject under study' and 'a keen understanding of what aspects of the self are the most important filters through which one perceives the world and, more particularly, the topic being studied' (p. 13). In telling my 'story', I aim to convey a sense of my positioning in relation to this project; a personal perspective on my epistemological and ontological assumptions that will serve as a context for the reflexive stance I aim to take throughout the book.

In the introductory chapter to *Disrupted Lives: how people create meaning in a chaotic world*, Becker[30] tells her own stories of living with disruption, and of how, despite being trained in an era where objectivity was the main goal and principal value of the social sciences, she realised that personal experience was at the heart of her intellectual interests. She writes, 'My studies of disruption in people's lives have been fuelled by my lifelong efforts to create a sense of continuity in my own life' (p. 8). She gives three reasons for telling her own stories: firstly, they illustrate the social and cultural context of disruption; secondly, her experience of asthma in which she 'felt the chaos of disruption at a visceral bodily level' sensitised her to the embodied nature of distress and the social constraints that 'heighten the difficulty people have in giving voice to bodily disruptions'[31] (p. 11); and thirdly, her story 'contained certain elements of narratives of disruption' that appeared in others' stories, thus conferring a personal 'moral authority'[32] (p. 12). I tell my own stories here in order to offer testimony, bear witness,[33] and take a kind of moral responsibility for my place in this book.

CUPBOARD UNDER THE STAIRS

On the day I started to write this account of my research journey, Tony, my husband, had decided to empty the cupboard under the stairs in order to gain access to the stair above, which needed repair. This involved removing the drawers from a filing cabinet in there. As I sorted through the contents, I found the files containing the handwritten first draft of my book about my illness. There were also envelopes packed with cards and letters, which had been sent to me around the time of my diagnosis and eventual surgery. As I looked through the messages of love and support, I could hardly bear to be reminded of that time—for the sadness and fear it all evoked, and for the tears that flowed. It seemed a strange and arbitrary (though perhaps synchronistic) reminder of just how far away from that world of illness, with all its uncertainty and contingency, I can feel ... and yet how powerful are the waves of memories that sweep me back into such desolation and loss. I think it was important for me to be reminded of that sense of devastation, for I have come to realise that, although mourning lies in the shadows of my illness story, paradoxically, I can 'forget' the consuming, soul-shrinking feeling of being cast into that 'other' world.

As I think back over the time from starting a PhD to the moment of writing this chapter, and wonder how to place my story in relation to the other stories in this book, it seems indeed synchronistic to be reminded of the 'peripeteia'[34] (a term used by Aristotle to refer to the occurrence of the unexpected on which the plot of a story hinges), which set in motion my own identity transformations; for it has been the sharing of common ground and mutual understandings with Jan, Jim, Pat and Yasmin that has touched me so profoundly. I have come to realise just how much my own struggles in the world of sickness and disability have not only provided an important reference point for me, but also a means of connection and communion with my co-participants that have, I hope, enhanced the quality of those relationships and the project as a whole.

I started my training as a counsellor in 1990 and was particularly drawn to the work of Carl Rogers on the person-centred approach to therapy. Rogers' ideas and values were close to my heart. I found his conversations with Polanyi and Buber[35] intellectually stimulating, but also profoundly meaningful and moving. I felt 'at home' with Rogers' trust in people, and with his view that, given the right conditions, we each have the capacity to find our own way forward; that our 'inner experience is a precious resource to be drawn upon and trusted'[36] (p. 174).

When I re-read *A Way of Being* some eight years later, his words, 'we are wiser than our intellects'[37] (p. 106), particularly caught my attention. And this was entirely selective: a very conscious projective identification. I was drawn to the phrase because the events of the intervening years had given me a particular reference point and personal insight into its meanings. Frank[38] describes his book *The Wounded Storyteller* as 'put together out of my need to make sense of my own survival' (p. xiii). This book springs from my own comparable need to find meaning and purpose in my own illness experience.

ILLNESS STORY

In 1993, I developed a tingling/pins-and-needles sensation on the left side of my face, which spread down my left arm. I saw my general practitioner (GP), was referred to a neurologist and admitted to hospital for tests. These revealed that I had a swelling deep down in the lower right thalamic region of my brain, at the top of the brain stem. Radiography suggested that it could be either a haemorrhagic tumour or a malformed cluster of blood vessels—a kind of 'birthmark'—which had lain dormant for the first 40 years of my life, but had then haemorrhaged within itself and swollen. I was told that it was too deep-seated for surgery; that the risks of removal or even biopsy were too great; it was therefore decided to monitor it through regular computerised tomography (CT) and magnetic resonance imaging (MRI) scans.

Over the next few months it continued to slowly haemorrhage and enlarge, and I lost all strength on my left side. By this time it was clearly and imminently life-threatening. There were two options, the first of which was radiosurgery, which

I was informed might delay its progression but would not cure it. The second option was a craniotomy, with the initial aim of biopsy and the very slim possibility of removal. The risks of surgery were high and included severe left-side disability and death. During that period of coming face to face with my mortality, a friend sent me a card on which were written the words of 14th century mystic Julian of Norwich,[39] a woman whose theology was of unconditional love and tenderness, compassion and hope. She wrote of how all things shall be well; I would say her words to myself, try to hold onto hope … hope that became increasingly slender as the cluster of blood vessels deep inside my brain continued to haemorrhage slowly, and to enlarge millimetre by millimetre. In the days leading up to the surgery, I knew that in medical terms my chances of survival were slim. There was a strong possibility of dying during the operation, but without it I would certainly have died. I can still find no words to express the fear and despair I felt as I looked at Tony and the children with the knowledge that I was likely to be separated from their lives. And yet, just before the operation, while fully experiencing the knowledge that I could die, I came increasingly and paradoxically to know that I would live. This was an intuitive knowledge beyond words, a sensing on the edge of my awareness. It felt deeply spiritual and transcended everything that was going on around me. This 'still small voice' was within me and beyond me. It was a certainty unlike anything I have ever known that, as events escalated, I was heading in the right direction and that I would live. Surgery would be done stereotactically; this meant having a steel frame screwed into my skull that day before the operation. The frame, together with the scanned images, allowed the surgeon to negotiate, to the millimetre, the path through my brain and to attempt the precise excision of the swelling.

The angioma was successfully removed and to the surprise of many, including some hospital staff, I made what was described as a remarkable recovery. I remain with a left-side disability: perpetual tingling, pain and impaired sensation on that side. However, my level of disability is considerably less than expected, and I am 'lucky' to be alive. Two days before my surgery I underwent a procedure that somehow seemed to sum up and encapsulate the complex and paradoxical nature of the whole experience. The test, known as a Wada Test, is to determine which side of the brain is dominant for speech and memory. In right-handed people, the left hemisphere is dominant, whereas in left-handed people, as I was at the time, either side can be dominant for these functions. This information would enable the surgeon to work out the path through my brain that least threatened these functions. After electroencephalography (EEG) wires were attached to my head and connected to a machine, a barbiturate drug, sodium amytal, was injected into the femoral artery, and then directed into the cerebral arteries, shutting down each side of the brain in turn. What I experienced was something that might be loosely called an 'altered state of consciousness'. What it actually felt like was being very pleasantly drunk. When I came to write about the experience later, I realised just how full of paradox and contradiction it had been:

Central to this was the feeling that at that point of facing my possible death, I felt so alive and, increasingly that I was going to live. Confined in a dark oppressive room and wired up to machines, I felt liberated and free to be myself. At my weakest and most vulnerable, I felt strong. As helpless as I had ever been in my life, I experienced some sense of power and control. In a state that was passive, I felt active, an agent not a victim. Lying there in a position of indignity, I found I had dignity. It was a time of contrasts and incongruity. At the centre of such precision and order, in the midst of science and technology, lay a redeeming sense of anarchy and chaos. Among the hard, impersonal machines and the menacing black metal, there was human warmth and good humour: the profoundly personal co-existed with the impersonal. Hope lived with fear.[40] (p. 107)

John O'Donohue[41] writes of the importance of paradox and contradiction as 'a creative force within the soul' (p. 148). I hope that I bring this acceptance and welcoming of paradox into my research relationships. I know that I am not afraid of despair or vulnerability. I know this because when I fully experience and express my own despair, I find hope, and when I fully experience and express my vulnerability, I find strength.

DISABILITY STORIES

The Body Silent,[42] a compelling account of a progressive spinal tumour and resulting quadriplegia written by anthropologist Robert Murphy, powerfully shows how serious illness and disability can rupture and alienate someone from the person s/he had previously been. In this 'extended anthropological field trip' (p. ix), he reflects on the impact of his 'quite remarkable illness upon my status as a member of society'. He vividly portrays the impact of a body that can no longer be taken for granted, and the resulting assault on his sense of self as an embodied and social being.

My own experience of illness and disability was similarly one of being thrown into disarray, of losing connection with the person I thought I was, as well as losing confidence in myself as a social being. I felt separated from the person I had been, wrenched from my life and from any sense that I had a life at all. I had no idea of where I was positioned in the world. In the early days after my surgery I was just grateful to be alive, to have some glimmer of hope that I might see my children grow up, to spend time with my family; I was glad to see sunshine and feel rain. But when that initial relief had faded—as it does—I started to feel the losses, and the guilt that I should experience loss at all. 'You're so lucky to be alive,' people would say. 'Don't you treasure every day?' And I would say, 'Yes, I do.' But I would grieve for the loss of taking for granted the 'taken-for-granted'. And I felt guilty for feeling so miserable. I should be grateful, and I was. I felt such joy to be able to meet my children from school, to be free to participate in the lives of my family. I was 'lucky', and I *felt* lucky; but why did I feel so sad? As I look back on that time, I realise that my sadness resided in my sense that I 'did not have a life'. I realise now how devastating the impact of it all was on my sense of myself as a person with identity, meaning and purpose. Oh yes, as a woman, I was a wife and a mother, and I was truly grateful that I could still fulfil those roles and be part of those relationships, but inside I felt that I was defined only in relation to others in my life. I could appreciate the miracle that was everyday life, but at the same time, struggle to feel that every minute of every day was precious. I would consciously reject the cliché that life-threatening illness helps one recognise the wonder of life but still felt the pressure of the dominant 'lucky to be alive' storyline.

In the years since then, I have at times felt like I am clawing my way out of a slippery-sided pit. I would get so far, then slide back down again. There were times when I could not imagine finding strength or the means to emerge. But sustained by my family and friends, it was possible. I told my story to friends and to counsellors. I knew I had lost any sense of myself as an independent person, and I could not imagine how I could ever find that again. I felt alone. How could anyone understand the feeling of being so close to death, of being prepared for dying, yet having the slender knowledge that I would live: and live with the most tenuous understandings of the effects and implications of my brain injury.

TURNING POINTS: A READING AND WRITING STORY

A turning point for me during the first few months of my recovery was reading Oliver Sacks' *A Leg to Stand On*, his autobiographical account of a serious leg injury and the effects of this on his peripheral nervous system; this caused him to lose sensation in the leg and his sense of proprioception, or the feeling of the leg as belonging to him. The effects of these losses led him to experience a profound disturbance to his sense of self and a resulting 'elemental anxiety and horror'[43] (p. 73). Here was some explanation of the impairment I was experiencing on my left side, the disruption to sensation and 'knowledge' of the exact location of my left arm. Here was an explanation of why it was so difficult to write with my previously dominant left hand. In addition, he wrote of the difficulty of being not only physically prostrate, but 'morally' so. Here was a neurologist who acknowledged and understood how difficult it was to undergo 'the realities of admission, the systematic de-personalisation that goes with becoming a patient' (p. 28). Here was a doctor who appreciated the complexity of being cast into the role of 'all-passive patient' (p. 122), who understood the ambiguity of such dependency on medical staff, where we can experience the 'cherished infant status' (p. 128) of being cared for, alongside acute anxiety over loss of control and independent status.

Oliver Sacks' book was a blessing to me because, in a sense, it 'gave me permission', as well as inspiration, to write. Exactly a year after my initial diagnosis, I needed to commemorate that day for myself, and tentatively tried to write about it. With considerable difficulty, I scrawled a few notes with my left hand. But the sensory disturbance on my left side as well as the impairment to my fine motor control meant that I could neither feel nor control the pen. Over the next few months I produced further scrawlings in the form of rather incoherent scraps of memories and feelings. But in February 1995, exactly a year after my neurosurgery, I felt the need to work through the experience in a more detailed and systematic way: the drive to engage creatively with it all was growing stronger, and I decided to try using my right hand. I was still relatively housebound at that time and limited as to what I was able to do, and so writing gave me something constructive to focus on, something that would engage my feelings and my intellect, but could also be done at home. Writing gave me a transitional space between my inner reality and the outside world, which at that stage still seemed very daunting. As a convalescent, I was still not quite ready for the 'bustling, callous, careless hugeness of the world'[44] (p. 127). So to stay at home and write gave me a space where I could negotiate my position in the world.

As I came to engage more deeply and more systematically in the writing, it became, as Oliver Sacks terms it, an 'inner journey' (personal communication). I found that I needed to re-enter the experience in order to recreate it. In re-experiencing the flow of feelings from the previous year, in empathising with myself, and connecting with my 'felt-sense' (a term used by Gendlin[45] to describe a sensation which lies on the edge of our awareness between the known and the unknown), I came to discover more about the journey it had been; to recognise, in Geertz' words, 'the connectedness of things that seem to have happened: pieced-together patternings, after the fact'[46] (pp. 2–3). Also, it was through that process that I came to realise that writing was not just an expression of something already known, but a means and process of discovery in itself—a realisation I came to in a poem[47] I wrote towards the end of 1996:

Raging Torrent
I crashed through the rapids
was swept along by the swirling torrent
bashed and battered by each rock
slashed by its razor-edge
tossed into the air

Breathless, I came smashing down
in terror and exhilaration
carried along by the force of the current
pulled down by the undertow into recesses dark and bleak

But moving, always moving in the right direction
the only direction

There was no choice

It was my river
the course I was on
a journey of the soul
I knew it
but I did not know that I knew it

Not until later
when I revisited the rapids

Then I travelled slowly
studied each rock
considered its shape
examined its sharp edges
turned it over
saw the strata
the sub-strata

As I gazed into the depths
looked long and hard into the eddying whirlpools
I saw the connections
the strata that linked each rock

Then I recognised what was there all along
what I had seen on that first turbulent passage
what I had registered, but at a level
beyond conscious awareness

The need to make conscious what was unconscious
to see the connections
in order to come to know
what I know
to find meaning
in the memory

Writing enabled me to explore, to discover connections, and to find order and meaning in the experience, or perhaps, in some existential sense, to impose order and meaning as a way of gaining some sense of control over a situation in which I had been essentially powerless; to claim something from it rather than be claimed by it. Reflecting on it all enabled me to integrate intellect and feeling as a way of making sense and finding value in an experience that had been lived 'in the moment'. Over that year, I wrote an account of the whole experience, which developed into a book.[48]

Herndl,[49] in a review of cancer autobiographies, writes: 'The problems of ethical storytelling involve writers' attitudes toward how they will use their newly gained senses of self and community to translate a physical experience into an ethical one' (p. 222) and observes that they 'share with most narratives the deep need to make some sort of meaning out of experience, to find a point or purpose to suffering' (p. 224).

Arthur Frank[50] identifies three types of illness narrative: restitution stories that are 'about the triumph of medicine'; chaos stories in which 'the suffering is too great for a self to be told'; and quest stories in which 'the meaning of the journey emerges recursively: the journey is taken in order to find out what sort of journey one has been taking' (p. 117). In retracing the steps of my own journey, I found out more about what kind of journey it had been, and in re-creating that journey, I found my voice, my 'embodied presence' (p. 145) as a storyteller.

In writing an essentially self-contained story with a beginning, middle, and end, I was making sense of the experience while giving it shape and form. However, I agree with Frank when he describes quest stories as risking romanticising illness. He writes, 'The risk of quest stories is like the risk of the Phoenix metaphor: they can present the burning process as too clean and the transformation as too complete' (p. 135). I am aware that my own quest story with its 'neat and tidy' ending hides the fact that I still live in the shadow of a life-threatening condition. I still have symptoms that on occasion require investigation, and when I return to the hospital for tests, I fear 'going back into' that world of 'being disconnected from my daily life, and from the lives of those around me'[51] (p. 354). So my self-contained quest story was inevitably 'too clean' and could only be *part* of the story.

While I wanted and needed that part of the story to be heard, I was aware that it was a difficult story for others to hear. By telling it in written form, I was offering people the choice of whether to read it, or not, or to choose which parts to read. For example, I knew it was difficult for people to hear about the stereotactic frame screwed into my head. (I also knew how much it meant to me when people could hear about it without turning away.) By describing it in writing, I was inviting responses, but also keeping myself safe in the sense that I could avoid their discomfort or rejection of me as someone who had experienced what Frank[52] describes as the 'unspeakable' (p. 355). Experiencing the unspeakable involves being placed in the position of 'object', of becoming, as a patient, 'an instance of this or that category to get done' (p. 361). This objectification is not only a loss of agency, but of personhood. In Buber's terms,[53] it is the 'I-It' relationship (1937).

Writing was a way in which I could attempt to express the 'unspeakable', and regain a sense of agency, as well as a means of making my voice heard. White and Epston[54] suggest that in many circumstances, particularly in the Western world, 'writing achieves unsurpassed authority from the fact that it is not heard but seen' (p. 34). In putting a personal account into the public domain and in offering my story as a written contribution to 'conversations' with the medical establishment, I was inviting responses. Anatole Broyard[55] writes of the need to personify his illness, and of wanting 'to be a good story' for his doctor (p. 25). I look back at that time when I first started to write, and realise that I wanted 'them' to know that this was what it was like. It meant a great deal to me when my surgeon, after reading the manuscript of the book, asked me how it had felt to face the prospect of my death. In acknowledging his sense of the unknown and his positioning as a doctor, he was silently acknowledging his own mortality, risking something of himself, and offering his humanity. Jellinger[56] who reviewed my book in the *European Journal of Neurology* described it as giving a 'perceptive and vivid view of a patient's life in hospital' that would 'offer valuable aid to healthcare professionals and counsellors alike' (p. 434). The fact that I received responses and generated further conversations with doctors who had contributed to my care, and from others who had read my account, was important to me and gave me a sense not only of resisting the diagnostic identity that medicine bestows, but also of having made a small contribution to the 'mosaic' of illness experience.

GENESIS OF RESEARCH IDEA

In 1998, I returned to my training as a counsellor; it felt right. I knew I had the potential to form relationships that were reciprocal and healing. I loved the reconnection with the ideas and values of Carl Rogers and Martin Buber. I appreciated the intellectual as well as affective engagement this kind of work gave me. When I read John McLeod's *Narrative and Psychotherapy*,[57] it had a major impact on me, and it was through this that I was introduced not only to narrative approaches to therapy, but also to the wealth of ideas exploring storytelling, the nature of reality, the concept of the person and the relationship between selfhood and culture. I loved the interdisciplinary roots of narrative ideas. I had been what was termed an 'all-rounder' at school; reasonably able at a broad range of subjects, though not particularly strong in any one field. But, excited and stimulated by these ideas, I tentatively dipped my toe in the water of more academic writing. In 1999, I had the opportunity to write a paper for an 'Auto/Biography' conference at Southampton University entitled 'Marginal Lives and Mainstream Concerns', and relished the prospect of writing on issues that were broadly sociological but would draw on my autobiographical writing and reading as well as on my developing interest in narrative ideas. In the paper, which was later published in *Auto/Biography*,[58] I set out to examine the factors within society and within the hospital setting which can have a marginalising effect on the person who is ill. I also explored the ambiguity and contradictions of being a patient. To illustrate and substantiate my points, I drew on my own story[59] and also on Sacks' *A Leg to Stand On*.[60] I found that working on the paper was a way of taking a step back and examining my experience from a greater distance and a wider angle. I was still making sense of it, but situating it more broadly in its social context: it was my experience with all of its uniqueness, subjectivity and partiality, but it also represented the experience of being a member of a particular group that is positioned as patients.

In addition, the paper offered me an opportunity to explore and reflect on my own writing process. Frank,[61] writing of illness, uses the analogy 'narrative wreckage': of being 'ship-wrecked by the storm of the disease'; he views storytelling as a way through this wreckage where 'a self is being formed in what is told' (p. 55). Although I knew from my experience as counsellor and as client that telling stories is healing, writing enabled me to learn 'firsthand' (an interesting metaphor, as my right hand had become my first hand) that it is also creative of the self; as Potts[62] writes in 'Narratives of the Self', a paper looking at the function of narrative in the re-construction of self after breast cancer, it is, 'by and through the narrative process that the self, and new selves, are established against the threats and changes that disease brings' (p. 27). All of this came to inform my research methodology.

In a paper considering creativity from the perspective of Donald Winnicott, Day Sclater[63] argues that the products of creativity occupy the same psychic space as the transitional comfort objects of infancy; and so, stories similarly occupy the ground between internal and external reality, connection and separation, self and non-self. She writes, 'Making sense by telling stories facilitates also the making of self' (p. 89). I see the early stages of my struggle to write as the beginning of a process not of the reconstruction of a fixed sense of self, but as a conscious engagement in the evolutionary process of becoming, and of transformation. Carl Rogers[64] views creativity as the 'emergence in action of a novel relational product, growing out of the uniqueness of the individual on the one hand, and the materials, events, people or circumstances of life on the other' (p. 351). He continues: 'the mainstream of creativity seems to be the same tendency which we discover so deeply as the curative force in psychotherapy—man's tendency to actualize himself, to become his potentialities' (p. 351).

LOSS AND TRANSFORMATION

In his introduction to *An Anthropologist on Mars*,[65] Oliver Sacks writes of how disease 'can play a paradoxical role, by bringing out latent powers, developments, evolutions … that might never be seen, or even imaginable, in their absence' (p. xii) and tells the stories of people whose neurological conditions have profoundly changed their lives, and for whom such transformations have involved creation as well as loss and dissolution. The paradox of illness stories is that they can encompass loss, chaos and meaninglessness alongside order, creative transformation and meaning-making. Such metamorphoses inform and shape our lives; they take us into territories where we recreate ourselves and yet return to mourning.

For example, one of my previous conceptions of self was thrown into complete disarray by my illness and subsequent left-side disability. I am no longer a left-handed person. I have 'learnt' to write with my right hand, and after 14 years I can manage fairly well. There are things that I can no longer do; I can't carry a cup of coffee in my left hand without spilling it, and I have trouble using a knife and fork.

I can use my left hand for gross motor functions such as carrying a bag, but, because I can't feel what I am holding, I may drop it unless I look to ensure it is still in my hand. When sociologist and writer Ann Oakley fractured her right arm, she reflected on issues of embodiment and identity, and wrote of 'the cultural dominance of right-handedness'[66] (p. 47). The Latin word for left is 'sinister', with its negative connotations, and in French it is 'gauche', with associations of clumsiness, whereas the Latin word for right is 'dexter', with associations of dexterity and skill. But I was happy to be left-handed; and of course now that I am no longer left-handed I am in fact extremely clumsy. I have lost count of the number of times I have burnt my left hand when cooking, or dropped glasses, jars and crockery on the kitchen floor—forgetting to use my eyes to ensure I was holding something properly with my left hand.

Associated with my left-handedness, and certainly with being able to use both hands, was my musical self. I had grown up in a 'musical house': both my parents played piano, and as a child, I had learnt to play. As a teenager in the late 60s/early 70s, I took up the guitar. It was the era of the singer-songwriter: Jackson Browne, Leonard Cohen, Bob Dylan, Carole King, Joni Mitchell and James Taylor. I loved to sing. The piano and guitar enhanced my work as a teacher in Birmingham, and when I taught in Zambia, I took my guitar with me: my students taught me African songs, and I taught them English and American songs. Two years before my illness, I had started to learn the saxophone: it was an expressive instrument that felt like an extension of my voice, and it suited me immediately. I was drawn to its beauty, its clear mellow sound, and the strength and subtlety of its tone. My musical self and my associations with it of freedom and voice seemed to disintegrate when I could no longer play those instruments. My writer sense of self, then, has developed out of, and in response to, the experience of illness and loss. It has become an important source of meaning and identity for me, and a place where I can reclaim the sense of independence I had previously found in making music.

When I see MRI scans of my brain, in one cross-section there is a black hole from the angioma that bled and was removed, and in another, there is the perfect circle of another angioma: a time-bomb possibly ticking away. I feel both the fear that is evoked and a sense of being on the edge of chaos, as well as an intuitive, tacit knowing that tells me it won't happen again. But it is very much part of who I am now and as such is 'incorporated' into my identity in the Latin sense of *in corpore*. And so, as a person whose sense of self now includes writing and research, I am not only writing *about* illness but *with* and through a differently embodied sense of myself, therefore reclaiming and regaining my association with my body.

LOOKING OUTWARDS

Through my work in counselling, I came to know four other people who had undergone different forms of major surgery, and as I heard their stories, the seed of an idea began to germinate. I became curious about others' experiences of illness and began to think about the possibility of working in a person-centred way to hear and to participate in the telling of such stories. I had worked with my own story and also felt a connection to, and interest in, the stories of others whose lives had been affected, disrupted and irrevocably transformed by illness: a sense of common ground as well as awareness of the unique nature of each person's story. My interest in exploring others' stories was in a sense part of my own journey of discovery and transformation, but was also a way of reaching out and working with others. My identity transformations had led me to discover writing as a place of exploration, discovery and creation—and vice versa—my writing had led to my own identity transformations. The 'inner journey' was leading outwards; the individual story was part of a more collective narrative. Just as the consciousness-raising of the women's movement in the 1970s gave political significance to personal experience, so the shared and collective illness story affirms the mutuality and community of those who are ill. And it was in this recognition of illness as shared social experience that I started to wonder whether there might be the potential here for a research project—maybe even a PhD. I then wrote to and talked with potential research supervisors about my ideas and was put in touch with Kim Etherington at Bristol. The 'fit' between Kim's considerable experience in narrative inquiry, as well as her interests in trauma and reflexivity, and my own personal and intellectual interests led me to apply formally to the University of Bristol for a place as a research student with Kim as my supervisor.

The period of writing and reflection that I have recounted here had a direct bearing on the evolution of my research methodology; I consider this in more detail in Part 3.

STORIES OF DISABILITY, LIBERATION AND INDEPENDENCE

In 2003, I started my study for a PhD at the University of Bristol. Since I live in Birmingham, this would require me to travel. I initially registered as a part-time MPhil/PhD student. As is usual within the United Kingdom, I would be required to complete training courses and assessments in research methods and also to upgrade my research project from MPhil to PhD. At the age of 49, nine years after surviving serious brain injury and living with the resulting disabilities, this felt terrifying as well as exciting and potentially liberating. I was sure that I wanted to do this; I knew exactly the focus of my research; I understood very clearly why I was so interested in and connected to illness narratives. I was motivated, passionate and curious about the area I would be investigating, as well as delighted to find a context in which I could write; it was a means of combining my academic and personal interests. I had a sense of the kind of methodology to which I was drawn. I knew I had the qualities and experience to work with people in such a way as to facilitate the telling of illness stories. But I had no idea at all how I would cope with the demands of travelling, carrying books, my total lack of computer skills and the difficulty of writing with my non-dominant right hand. I was worried by my visual-spatial difficulties. I had constant pain on my left side.

So, full of trepidation, panic, uncertainty, excitement, doubt and questions, I set out for Bristol. I would register, meet my supervisor for the first time (having only been in telephone contact prior to that) and have an introductory session on using the library facilities. It all sounded straightforward. I would use the long train journey there to prepare myself. I knew I would struggle with finding my way around, but I would take a taxi to the university and ask for help if I needed it. I was a mature, independent woman, I reminded myself. In my journal, I wrote:

> What a tornado of doubts and panic. Is this a huge mistake? Am I doing the right thing? Am I clever enough? Do I have the energy? The intellect?' Is my health up to this? Am I pushing myself too hard?

I found that first trip to Bristol hugely daunting. I was terrified that I was taking on too much and that the demands of the venture would threaten my health. While I was aware that my disabilities were relatively minor in terms of the kind of brain injury I had sustained, I feared that they would put the whole project out of my reach. The relatively invisible nature of my disabilities is such that they are not immediately identifiable. In a short account of my experience as a student with disabilities who was embarking on a PhD, I wrote:

> If you were to look at me, I do not think you would see disability. If you were to spend some time with me, you would see that sometimes my concentration wanders; you might see my engagement and enthusiasm, but you would also see me disengaging with tiredness in my eyes. If you were to observe me walking, you would see my left side moving more slowly than my right, sometimes dragging, sometimes bumping into things on the left. You might notice my left hand moving like a mechanical grabber, the kind you saw in 'fun fairs' in the 60s, awkward and clumsy ... [67] (p. 195)

My main anxiety was how I would be able to fulfil the requirements of a PhD when I had no computer skills whatsoever; I could not imagine being able to manipulate a computer mouse or type with my non-dominant right hand.

Illness had disrupted my sense of myself as a social being. I had lost confidence, and did not quite feel fully part of the world. However, although I felt very vulnerable I also knew that if I could express that vulnerability and have it truly received, then it would be transforming and I would find my own strength. In my journal, I wrote:

> It is in the tension between the knowing and the not knowing, between the fragility and the strength, the hopeless and the hopeful, the giving in and the carrying

on, the retreat and going forward; if I express and am understood, I can go on. I can take the risk, I will 'feel the fear, and do it anyway'. It is a huge effort - both physical and emotional to go to Bristol - but I also see my learning and development (as researcher) as being about relationships. They are central to me, to my sense of self. Belonging, being accepted, finding stimulation, affirmation and validation activate my own capacity for discovery and creativity (as well as my capacity to engage with others in a way which is affirming)[68] (p. 196).

FEBRUARY 2003

I found the first research-training unit exhilarating and exciting, but I was so utterly exhausted that it frightened me. When I'm very tired (and sometimes when I'm not very tired) I have visual/spatial difficulties, my reading slows down and I have difficulty finding my way around new places. It was an intensive three-day course with reading and preparation each night for the next day; my eyes were sore from the physical struggle of reading. The first evening, I was so tired I could barely think and became terribly lost on my way back to where I was staying. I am unable to run, and so, alone and disorientated in the dark, I stumbled down a bank with trees. I felt completely helpless but tried to stay calm. After some time, I found my way back to the security gate, and asked to be shown the way to my accommodation. I was distressed and felt humiliated. They gave me directions but I was unable to visualise the way. When I asked to be escorted, they clearly thought I was stupid. And I felt stupid. Stupid and frustrated that my brain was no longer able to cope with getting around easily in the ordinary world. When I eventually arrived back in my room, I rang home and burst into tears. I tried to do some preparatory reading for the next day, but I had such a feeling of intense pressure in my head that I struggled to focus on the text. I was very frightened and concerned about getting lost. Was I pushing myself too hard? Was I risking another haemorrhage? I checked the strength on my left side. It seemed to be all right, but I knew I would have to be careful, and that I should monitor my symptoms. I also decided it would be wise to talk to my neurologist once I was home.

I saw someone at the disability/access unit who advised me to apply for Disabled Students Allowance. This would involve having my needs assessed, and I felt this would be helpful as a means of clarifying my needs. At that stage I was dependent on the goodwill of family and friends to type my handwritten scrawl. I knew it would be some time until my needs assessment, but in the meantime I happily engaged with the reading and the assignment writing. And as I worked, my confidence grew. While I felt it was important to have my difficulties acknowledged, I would not let them prevent me from doing what I was capable of. I felt a huge 'neurological' drain on my energy, but I also knew that I did not have to accept a 'language of deficit'[69] (p. 353).

When I told my neurologist about my symptoms – the feeling of pressure in my head, the increase in tingling on my left side, and the extreme exhaustion – I half expected, or rather hoped, that he would say, 'Don't waste my time'. I was shocked when he said, 'In the light of your history, we'll do an EEG and an MRI scan.' He told me not to overdo it. I knew from experience that it would be a while before the appointment came through, so I tried to put it to the back of my mind. In my journal, I wrote:

> I'm shocked. As I go over the appointment in my head, as I process it all, things he said start to emerge: 'It's nearly ten years. You've done really well.' I know I have, but implicit in that statement is the idea that I was not expected to live this long - that 10 years is better than expected.

> He told me he would be retiring on June 20th, said he hadn't envisaged it - suggested it was to do with changes in NHS. I wished him well and said I was sorry that he was going before he had planned to, and in this way. I feel a huge sense of loss; a person of his wisdom, humanity and experience will be really missed, and not just by his patients, but also by his colleagues.

Those early months in Bristol were very much a time of feeling my way, of finding reference points. Although I felt 'blocked' initially by my anxieties and fears, I was spurred on by my drive towards independence and the potential for the realisation of a new sense of self. My strong feeling that there was something meaningful and 'right' about the path I was on, that everything we experience in life is part of the process that leads us to where we are and who we are now, was echoed in a phrase in Coelho's book *The Alchemist*[70] when the traveller Santiago meets the alchemist who tells him, 'Everything you need to know, you've learnt through your journey'.

JUNE 2003

My experience of 'needs assessment' in relation to my disabilities and my EEG appointment proved to be an illuminating part of that journey: there was a marked contrast in the way each was carried out—a contrast that highlights some subtle differences in relation to knowledge and power. I found the disability needs assessment a valuable and positive experience. It felt like it was the first time I could detail my specific difficulties and have them recognised and understood. At the same time, I felt that I was being related to as a person with capabilities and equal rights; this was not clichéd talk, but a genuine recognition of my rights to an independent life in which I would be able to do things for myself. It was straightforward and focused on identifying the effects of my medical condition and the impact of this on studying, and on determining my specific needs in relation to studying requirements, technology and materials that would enable me to carry out research. There was recognition of how my reliance on others to type my work restricted my independence. I greatly appreciated the way this assessment was carried out. It was not condescending, patronising or pathologising.

A few days later, in contrast to this, I had the EEG. After the electrodes had been attached to my scalp, the technician asked me lots of questions. Halfway through the EEG, he stopped and drew a diagram of the holes and crevices on my skull. This was fine; I understood its necessity. Then he asked a young woman, who was present because she was 'on work experience' in the department, if she wanted to feel my head. I felt like an object. She asked him questions about my EEG tracings, and as he answered them, he clearly did not want me to hear what was said; I sensed discomfort in his voice and something slightly evasive in his tone. So I asked my own questions: 'What does that mean?' 'You mentioned spiky patterns in that region; why is that significant?' 'Why did you say to her, "I'll tell you later?"'

I reflected on the experience later:

> I know when I'm in the position of patient and very anxious, I protect myself by engaging my intellect; it's an assertion of power when I feel helpless. I ask sharp and pertinent questions and push for answers. It is part of my need to be related to as a person. I hate the passivity of the patient role. I'm also aware that since it is my brain which is being investigated, I feel a strong need to show I can use it, and to show that it is not a physiological object - it is part of who I am. I understand that he is not supposed to comment, but I reserve the right to question someone who is sticking electrodes on my scalp and observing the patterns of electrical activity in my brain: who is talking *about* me, and not *to* me.

I was still waiting for an appointment for my MRI scan and would not get the results of the EEG until both tests were done. I carried on with my academic work, aware that this is part of the way I deal with the legacy of anxiety and uncertainty, and that my research is a way of acknowledging their presence while also maintaining a degree of distance.

The following week, I rang the MRI unit to ask if they could give me any indication of a date. I was told they had not received any 'paperwork'. I then rang Dr. A's secretary, who told me she had delivered the letter personally. 'In any case', she added, 'there's a 10 month waiting list.' I felt exhausted, helpless and anxious; I knew he would be retiring the following Friday, and I felt totally blocked by the secretary/gate-keeper and the bureaucracy of the system.

A week later I rang the MRI unit once more, to be told, yet again, that I was still not on the list, and that they had not received the paperwork. I rang his secretary again, and had the following conversation:

> 'I'm one of Dr. A's patients - I ...'
> 'You were', she interrupts, 'he's just retired.'
> 'I know that,' I snap. 'He told me. I'm ringing to inquire about the MRI he requested. The MRI Centre has still not received any paperwork.'

> *'Well, there's a 12 month waiting list ...' she insists. I think, 'I know, but I wouldn't mind being on it.' But I say, 'Can another duplicate be sent down?'*
> *'Well, I'll have to get the registrar to sign it.'*

I think of Arthur Frank's phrase: 'something else to get done'—or not, in this case—and of how any of us when we are positioned as patients can become invisible, and of how we can't be sure we won't get lost or overlooked as we disappear from view; a valuable reminder to me of the passive role we can be ascribed within a system where, in Foucault's terms,[71] the domains of knowledge and domains of power are inseparable.

Dr. A had told me that I could see my surgeon for my follow-up out-patient appointments, rather than a neurologist I did not know. So at that point I decided to ring the surgeon's secretary. Three days later, I received a date for my MRI scan. I finally had my scan; the results both of that and of my angiogram showed no significant change. They would see me again in two years' time.

The whole process was a reminder to me of how difficult it is for any of us to be in the position of patient, experiencing anxiety and helplessness within the 'system'. It also reminds me of the vital importance of relationships between healthcare practitioners and patients; a point Jerome Bruner makes when he tells the story of a nurse he encountered after an operation to remove cataracts. He tells of how through warmth and humour, she '*recognised* my human plight and shared it with me'[72] (p. 5), and writes of the importance of this recognition, and of how liberating it can be when we experience that understanding.

OCTOBER 2003

I struggled for a while with acquiring the computer skills I needed; my abiding memory of the IT training unit was one of ringing a friend and sobbing that I found it too difficult to type with my right hand and would have to give up my PhD because I would never be able to master the use of email, Internet and 'Word' documents. Over time my confidence has grown significantly in this area—although there are still times when I feel I am working at the edge of my IT capabilities.

I became used to my trips to Bristol. A particular turning point for me was the day I caught the bus rather than a taxi from Temple Meads, Bristol's central railway station, to the university. That day, there was a group of Welsh women who had, I think, come to Bristol for a day of shopping. It was a warm, sunny day and I remember sitting on the bus and feeling just the most lovely, liberating sense of being part of the ordinary world. In that most mundane of achievements, on a beautiful day, I felt joy in sitting on a bus amidst a group of warm, lively women, and a sense of independence that came from doing this 'all by myself'. I could be part of the world again.

I came to appreciate time on my own; at times I would feel adventurous and independent, while at other times I would feel like hiding away in my room. I liked being away from home, but I hated it too. I appreciated the solitude and time to pursue this new academic life, but I was also afraid of being away from home, of the distance and the sense of separation. I knew it was an echo of that awful fear of separation when it looked like I would die; that journey out of illness had to be a journey through this 'separation anxiety'. Serious illness can be an experience of regression, of return to child-like dependency. As I came to realise the extent of that, I knew that being in Bristol, though scary, was important and necessary, and that my pathway into research was also a step towards transformation.

I felt a strong sense of wanting to 'make a difference' and a hope that my research might illuminate understanding and challenge the 'results culture' of the NHS, where hospitals are given scores based on (among other criteria such as cleanliness and waiting times) 'deaths within 30 days after operations'.[73] I knew that in such a culture I was 'lucky' to have surgery at all; in fact, one of the doctors later told me that my operation was so risky that no other surgeon would have attempted it. I knew I was fortunate to have a surgeon with the confidence, the skill and the courage to take risks.

ILLNESS AND STIGMA

I am aware that my move into writing and research was influenced to a degree by my need to prove to myself and anyone who might doubt that my brain is still in working order. There is stigma attached to serious illness—we are somehow 'other'. Of course, there is a sense in which I am implicated in stigmatisation here; or else why would I need to prove to myself and to others that my brain is 'still in working order'? Couser[74] suggests that many first-person narratives of 'those who represent their own experiences with disability' are often 'consciously countering ignorance about or stigmatization of their conditions' and 'insofar as they initiate and control their own representation … their narratives may seek to *reduce* their vulnerability to pre-inscribed narrative' (p. 20). I certainly recognise this more 'political' motivation in my own decisions to write and research in the area of illness.

The stigmatisation associated with brain injury was clearly exemplified in the BBC programme 'Top Gear' in 2007: the presenter, Richard Hammond, was seriously injured following a crash when his jet-powered car came off a runway at 280 mph. Despite sustaining serious brain injury, he made a good recovery, but on his return to the show, Jeremy Clarkson, the main presenter, asked if he was 'mental', while co-presenter, James May offered him a tissue 'in case he started dribbling'. The handling of his return to the programme resulted in many complaints and was described by Peter McCabe, chief executive of the UK brain injury charity 'Headway', who said: 'This has created such anger among members of Headway. It really was offensive and insulting to all those people living with brain injuries'.[75]

Studies such as those by Simpson, Grahame, Mohr *et al.*,[76] exploring cultural variations in understandings of brain injury, and Swift and Wilson,[77] examining misconceptions surrounding brain injury, report substantial lack of awareness and understanding. Linden, Rauch and Crothers,[78] in a study focusing on public attitudes to brain injury, found that although the range of outcomes following brain injury is vast and depends on the interaction of many factors, the 'label of "brain injured" reduces the individual to a one-dimensional character with no real sense of personhood' (p. 1012).

Nevertheless, and perhaps rather naively, I was surprised to encounter stigmatising attitudes to brain injury 'closer to home' within the relatively 'sheltered' professional discourse of the university. In 2005, I attended a seminar on the way in which neuroscience can contribute to and inform teaching and learning within schools. The academic who reported on the project talked of the use of functional neuroimaging as a means of research into learning. In the course of the seminar, he referred to the brains of people who had experienced neurological injury such as strokes as being comparable to television sets that had been thrown from a third floor window and smashed, and whose wires were entangled and disconnected. I was shocked; initially I could not take in the use of such an analogy. I think it is probably fair to say that my heightened sensitivity to the use of the metaphor was connected with my own experience, though colleagues sitting nearby were also taken by surprise. I hope that I would have been equally taken aback even if I had not experienced brain injury. But I think it is a powerful example of the stigmatising attitudes associated not only with neurological damage but also with any serious illness.

I think the experience, though surprising, was useful as a way of sensitising me to stigmatising language and attitudes regarding illness, and thus has had an impact on my work. Sontag[79] powerfully demonstrates how the myths surrounding illness are embedded in and perpetuated by the metaphors we employ. I look at the use of figurative language and imagery associated with illness in Chapter Six.

SHARING THE PATH

My experience of inhabiting the world of illness, of living with a heightened sense of mortality, of being differently embodied, and of the search for meaning involved in this, has raised my awareness of the cultural context of illness stories, sensitised me to stories which go untold, and heightened my appreciation of the uniqueness of each person's story, all of which have affirmed for me a sense of what unites us as human beings. In telling my stories and venturing to create a space in which others can tell their stories, I am offering what Geertz[80] terms 'local knowledge' to complement the medical, scientific account of us as cases. For I recognise that both scientific and experiential, 'narrative' knowledge are necessary if we are to create fuller and richer pictures of human realities.

Personal stories, in the way they convey lived experience within a particular social context, play an important part in enriching and adding depth, texture and complexity to 'pictures of human reality'. Frank writes of 'thinking with' stories as something we do when we enter into another's story and allow our 'own thoughts to adopt the story's immanent logic of causality, its temporality and its narrative tensions'[81] (p. 18). We 'listen with' stories when we feel their power and allow that resonance. Indeed, it was feeling the power and resonance of Oliver Sacks' *A Leg to Stand On*[82] that enabled me to write my own story. My experience of the storytelling process has been that it is deeply reciprocal, connective and life affirming: it is to do with not only 'walking the path',[83] but *sharing* the path and flows from, in Buber's words, the '*a priori* of relation'[84] (p. 43). In others' responses to my story, and in being invited to hear or read the stories of others, I have been privileged to participate in what Buber terms the 'I of endless dialogue'[85] (p. 89). It is this reciprocal, mutual, dialogic nature of storytelling that has led me in the direction of researching others' illness narratives.

My journey was (and still is) one through which I am learning about the subtleties of disability and the effects of illness. I am discovering more about a topic that has personal resonance for me as well as gaining understanding of its wider social and cultural implications, and of issues of knowledge and power. This introduction, then, has been an attempt to set a context for my narrative research with Pat, Jan, Jim and Yasmin, and to make some of the links between my illness experience, my writing and my professional background in counselling. In the course of this book, I will pick up many of these threads in the literature to which I refer, and also in relation to the development of my methodology. Laurel Richardson[86] uses the image of a crystal (p. 934) to suggest the multi-dimensional nature of postmodern texts; and it is in the nature of a crystal, with its reflection and refraction, its symmetry and its substance, its depth and its complexity, that I offer this approach to narrative inquiry.

REFERENCES

1. Eliot TS. *Little Gidding. The Complete Poems and Plays.* London: Faber and Faber; 1969. p. 197.
2. Martin V. *Out of my Head.* Lewes: Book Guild; 1997.
3. Bochner A. Narrative's virtues. *Qualitative Inquiry.* 2001; 7(2): 138.
4. Becker G. *Disrupted Lives: how people create meaning in a chaotic world.* Berkeley and Los Angeles: University of California Press; 1999.
5. Behar R. *The Vulnerable Observer.* Boston, MA: Beacon Books; 1996.
6. Etherington K. *Trauma, the Body and Transformation.* London: Jessica Kingsley; 2003.
7. Etherington K. *Becoming a Reflexive Researcher: using our selves in research.* London: Jessica Kingsley; 2004.
8. Clough P. *Narratives and Fictions in Educational Research.* Buckingham: Open University Press; 2002.
9. Leitch R. *Journey into Paradox: re-searching unconscious in teacher identity using creative narrative.* Unpublished Ed. D. thesis, University of Bristol; 2003.
10. Ellis C. *Final Negotiations.* Philadelphia: Temple University Press; 1995.

11. Ellis C, Bochner AP. Autoethnography, personal narrative, reflexivity: researcher as subject. In: Denzin NK, Lincoln YK, editors. *Handbook of Qualitative Research*. London: Sage; 2000.
12. Sparkes A. The fatal flaw: a narrative of the fragile body-self. *Qual Inquiry*. 1996; 2(4): 463–94.
13. Ellis C. *The Autoethnographic 'I': a methodological novel about teaching and doing ethnography*. Walnut Creek, CA: Alta Mira; 2004.
14. Spry T. Performing auto-ethnography: an embodied methodological praxis. *Qualitative Inquiry*. 2001; 7: 706–32.
15. Leitch, op. cit.
16. Ellis, op. cit.
17. Ellis, Bochner, op. cit.
18. Etherington, op. cit. pp. 179–94.
19. Sparkes A. *Telling Tales in Sport and Injury*. Champaign: Human Kinetics; 2002.
20. Speedy J. *Narrative Inquiry and Psychotherapy*. Basingstoke: Palgrave Macmillan; 2008.
21. Spry, op. cit.
22. McLeod J. *Qualitative Research in Counselling and Psychotherapy*. London: Sage; 2001.
23. Church, K. *Forbidden Narratives: critical autobiography as social science*. London: Gordon and Breach; 1995.
24. Etherington, op. cit.
25. Wachowski A, Wachowski L, directors. *The Matrix* [Film] USA: Warner Brothers; 1999.
26. Gadamer H. *Truth and Method*. 2nd ed. London: Sheed and Ward; 1975.
27. McLeod, op. cit.
28. Moustakas C. *Heuristic Research: design, methodology and applications*. Thousand Oaks, CA: Sage; 1990.
29. Behar, op. cit.
30. Becker, op. cit.
31. Ibid.
32. Ibid.
33. Frank A. *The Wounded Storyteller: body, illness and ethics*. Chicago: University of Chicago Press; 1995.
34. Aristotle. *Poetics*. Heath M, translator. London: Penguin; 1996.
35. Kirschenbaum H, Henderson V, editors. *Carl Rogers: dialogues*. London: Constable; 1990.
36. Rogers CR. *A Way of Being*. Boston, MA: Houghton Mifflin; 1980.
37. Ibid.
38. Frank, op. cit.
39. Julian of Norwich. *Revelations of Divine Love*. London: Penguin Classics; 1998.
40. Martin V. *Out of my Head*. Lewes: Book Guild; 1997.
41. O'Donohue J. *Anam Cara*. London: Bantam Press; 1997.
42. Murphy R. *The Body Silent*. London: WW Norton; 1990.
43. Sacks O. *A Leg to Stand On*. Revised Edition. London: Picador; 1991.
44. Sacks, op. cit.
45. Gendlin E. *Focusing*. New York, NY: Everest House; 1978.
46. Geertz C. *After the Fact: two countries, four decades, one anthropologist*. Cambridge, MA: Harvard University Press; 1995.

47. Martin V. A person-centred perspective on the marginalising effects of illness and hospitalisation. *Auto/Biography.* 2000; **8**(1–2): 19–26.
48. Martin, 1997, op. cit.
49. Herndl DP. Our breasts, our selves: identity, community, and ethics in cancer auto-biographies. *Signs.* 2006; **32**(1): 222–44.
50. Frank, op. cit.
51. Frank A. Can we Research Suffering? *Qual Health Res.* 2001; **11**(3): 353–62.
52. Ibid.
53. Buber M. *I and Thou.* Edinburgh: T&T Clark; 1937.
54. White M, Epston D. *Narrative Means to Therapeutic Ends.* New York, NY: Norton; 1990.
55. Broyard A. *Intoxicated by My Illness and Other Writings on Life and Death.* New York, NY: Clarkson and Potter; 1992.
56. Jellinger K. Book Review: Out of my Head. *Eur J Neurol.* 1997; **4**: 434.
57. McLeod J. *Narrative and Psychotherapy.* London: Sage; 1997.
58. Martin, 2000, op. cit.
59. Martin, 1997, op. cit.
60. Sacks, op. cit.
61. Frank, op. cit.
62. Potts L. Narratives of the self: stories of breast cancer and identity. *Auto/Biography.* 2000; **8**(1–2): 27–32.
63. Day Sclater S. Creating the self: stories as transitional phenomena. *Autobiography.* 1998; **6**(1–2): 85–92.
64. Rogers CR. *On Becoming a Person.* Boston, MA: Houghton Mifflin; 1961.
65. Sacks O. *An Anthropologist on Mars.* London: Picador; 1995.
66. Oakley A. *Fracture: adventures of a broken body.* Bristol: The Policy Press; 2007.
67. Martin V. Stories of liberation and independence. In: Etherington K, editor. *Becoming a Reflexive Researcher: using our selves in research.* London: Jessica Kingsley; 2004. pp. 195–201.
68. Martin, ibid.
69. Gergen K. Therapeutic professions and the diffusion of deficit. *J Mind Behav.* 1990; **11**: 35368.
70. Coelho P. *The Alchemist.* London: HarperCollins; 1999.
71. Foucault M. *Power/Knowledge: selected interviews and other writings.* New York: Pantheon Books; 1980.
72. Bruner J. Narratives of plight: a conversation with Jerome Bruner. In: Charon R, Montello M, editors. *Stories Matter: the role of narrative in medical ethics.* New York, NY: Routledge; 2002.
73. http://news.bbc.co.uk/2/shared/bsp/hi/nhs_league_03/html/tables.stm
74. Couser T. Paradigms' cost: representing vulnerable subjects. *Lit Med.* 2005; **24**(1): 19–30.
75. http://news.bbc.co.uk/1/hi/health/6324129.stm (accessed 2 Feb. 2007).
76. Simpson G, Mohr R, Redman A. Cultural variations in the understanding of traumatic brain injury and brain injury rehabilitation. *Brain Inj.* 2000; **14**(2): 125–40.
77. Swift TL, Wilson SL. Misconceptions about brain injury among the general public and non-expert health professionals: an exploratory study. *Brain Inj.* 2001; **15**(2): 149–65.

78. Linden MA, Rauch RJ, Crothers IR. Public attitudes towards survivors of brain injury. *Brain Inj.* 2005; **19**(12): 1011–17.
79. Sontag S. *Illness as Metaphor.* New York, NY: Farrar, Strauss and Giroux; 1989.
80. Geertz C. *Local Knowledge: further essays in interpretive anthropology.* New York, NY: Basic Books; 1983.
81. Frank, op. cit.
82. Sacks, op. cit.
83. Wachowski, Wachowski, op. cit.
84. Buber, op. cit.
85. Ibid.
86. Richardson L. Writing: a method of inquiry. In: Denzin NK, Lincoln YK, editors. *Handbook of Qualitative Research.* London: Sage; 2000.

CHAPTER 2

Pat's story

INTRODUCTION

Pat had been a nurse for many years and was working as an experienced renal nurse when she was diagnosed with kidney failure. Within two years of her diagnosis, she needed dialysis. She continued to work as a nurse up to and during the time of her dialysis. This was followed just under two years later by a kidney transplant. Shortly after her transplant, she experienced serious heart problems that led to heart surgery. Her health problems have had a major impact on every dimension of her life. This raised particular difficulties in terms of being a patient at the same time and on the same unit where she worked. I was introduced to Pat by a colleague who worked in healthcare. After making initial phone contact, I sent her the information sheet, followed up with a phone call, and arranged an initial visit. As a nurse who had undergone renal failure, Pat had experienced a major disruption to her life and a profound upheaval to both her personal and professional identities.

IT CHANGES YOU … THE CORE OF YOU, ACTUALLY

I drive over to meet Pat for the first time, aware that the 'peripeteia',[1] which Bruner[2] describes as 'a sudden reversal of circumstances' (p. 5) that had precipitated her story constituted a particularly powerful occurrence of the unexpected in which her world had been turned upside down. As I find my way to her house, I think of the power of her words on the phone: 'It changes you, the core of you, actually. You're not the same person … the surface is healed, but underneath you're not … you're left in a kind of limbo afterwards. Especially when you've been through a life-threatening and life-changing illness …'

I pull onto her drive and tentatively knock. An auburn-haired woman with a broad smile opens the door and greets me. 'Viv? Hello!' We shake hands. 'It's lovely to meet you!' she exclaims. 'Do come in—I've got the kettle on. Would you like some coffee or tea?'

'It's lovely to meet you too, Pat. Coffee would be great, thanks.' She shows me into the living room–a warm and cosy space, the noise of traffic humming in the distance. As she goes off to make coffee, I take out the information sheet and consent form, which I intend to leave with her. When we had talked on the phone, I had suggested she might want to leave signing it until after we had met, when she could make a more fully informed decision about her involvement in this research. We had talked about the interview process and I intended to start our meeting by discussing this in more detail. However, it was clear as we sat down to talk that Pat was eager to tell me her story; so I decided to leave this until later. There was an ease in this initial meeting, something I had sensed would be the case from our telephone conversations.

EVERYTHING IS TURNED ON ITS AXIS

I take a sip of coffee and say, 'I know a little of your illness experience from our chats on the phone, and I'm wondering, if I didn't know anything about it, and you were to tell me the story from the beginning, how would you start?'

'It was a Monday. The day before, we'd been to the Valley Railway, where they've got steam engines … I remember this puff of smoke blew into my face. I didn't think anything of it, but the next day I woke up and my eyesight in one eye was cloudy; my vision was blurred. And every day it was getting worse. By the Friday I got a bit worried, so I went to see the optician. She said she'd refer me to a neurologist. At that point, I was quite calm. The neurologist said, "Right, I'll give you some steroids. I think it's stress, but it is one of the indications of MS". And I was upset … you look into the future and you're quite healthy at the time, you're doing your job and just pootling along. Then suddenly you're faced with a future in a wheel chair, incontinence and everything else that it entails, and you think, oh my god …'

'So the future you thought you were going to have has been completely changed?' I ask, my own recognition informing my question.

'Yes—destroyed in that word. And yet you sort of hold on to that bit of hope … then he said, "I'm just going to check the kidney function, and I'll do some blood tests." And when the results arrived, he said, "Oh my god, your cholesterol's sky high." And when my kidney function test came back, it was abnormal … The thing was, I was nursing dialysis patients–I was doing haemodialysis at the time, so I knew exactly what was happening. And the consultant—he was just joking—said, "You'd better pick up a burger and fries on the way." I said, "Well, there'll be no fries for me because of the implications of potassium."'

Pat's story takes me straight into the heart of her experience; she describes the events and locates them in time and place within the 'landscape of action'[3] (p. 14). And as she faces the unknown, and struggles with the shock of it all, she takes me into her 'landscape of consciousness': her feelings, thoughts and meanings. This is terrain that she knows so well as a nurse, and to which she now belongs as a patient: her future 'destroyed in that word'.

'We got there and I couldn't stop crying … all of a sudden I was a renal patient. I remember sitting in my bed and this patient across the way says, "Oh, it's not so bad, kidney failure. Once they sort you out you'll be as right as rain." And I said, "I'm a dialysis nurse. I know what kidney failure is!" I was quite sharp with her. It was just terrifying. You don't see the good part of it, you see the bad part; you see years of being dependent on a machine, dependent on drugs, having to curtail your diet. And from a nurse's point of view—it's not that nurses are unfeeling, but unless you've been there, you don't know what it's like.'

As a renal nurse, Pat knows the implications of her diagnosis, and the impact it will have on her life. As a patient she *feels* those implications; she has 'been there' and 'knows what it's like' from a different standpoint. I check my understanding of this with her:

'So once you're in that patient position, you look at it from a completely different viewpoint?'

'Yeah–totally; everything is turned on its axis.' She pauses, and in silence we reflect on the enormity of a world turned on its axis; a reversal of circumstance such that Pat's world is turned upside down.

She continues, 'It's just … you become … you're not a person … not what you were. You're a kidney patient. Your persona changes, and you're in that bed.'

The impact of diagnosis snatches away her 'persona', and replaces it with 'kidney patient' who is 'in that bed'. Her medical knowledge and understandings intensify this sense of disintegration and chaos and reinforce the dislocation between Pat, the nurse with an ordered life, and Pat, the patient whose body is thrown into disarray and disorder. While knowledge can give a sense of control, the body's inner knowledge, once revealed through illness, destroys that illusion of control. As Pat reflects on the enormity of her world turned on its axis, she moves from the first-person 'I'm a dialysis nurse' to the second-person 'you're not a person, you're a kidney patient', her language providing and reflecting the distance for which she longs. The complexity and ambiguity of being both a renal nurse and renal patient are important issues that I will return to in greater detail later in this chapter.

'They said it would be about five years before I needed dialysis …' she continues. 'But I was on it within two … by Christmas, I was really quite ill—I couldn't even brush my teeth without getting out of breath, and I felt so cold. Your body slows down the production of red blood cells and you become quite anaemic', she explains to me. 'And that affects your breathing; you feel quite cold because of the lack of oxygen in your blood. But they sorted that out and I went back to work.'

As Pat tells her story, she moves back and forth between using her patient voice and her nurse voice, the one informing the other.

DIALYSIS

'Then a week before my birthday in July, they said I'd have to go on dialysis. I felt quite well at the time, so it just came out of the blue! I was on dialysis within a couple of days—the level of toxins was just so high. I was still going to the loo–you *do*, because your kidneys overcompensate. I used to be so thirsty because I was passing so much urine, and so I was drinking so much. Your kidneys overcompensate, and they try and get rid of all the toxins.

'So the day before my birthday, I was on dialysis in the unit where I worked. They made it quite nice actually—they clubbed together and bought me some flowers,' she remembers.

'But it was just …' she falters. 'One patient always sticks out in my mind, a young lad in his early 20s. He'd gone to join the army reserves, and they did blood and urine tests and found something. He was on dialysis the next hour and he was a fit young man!' she exclaims. 'His body had got used to the toxins. He was in end-stage renal failure. And the *shock* on his face … he was very non-compliant with his treatment and his diet because he had no time to get used to it … it was just the *shock* on his face,' she repeats.

'So seeing that happen to him really brought you face to face with your own shock?' I ask.

'I think it was because I'd built up a relationship with him over his sessions. And the shock on his face—and I thought one minute you're well and the next minute … and when they took me into the room to be dialysed–I was at work, and they were going to dialyse me after work–I'd keep going past the room 'cos someone was getting it ready for me … and I thought, this can't be happening.'

As Pat tells this story, in all its power, with its myriad reflections of her own shock and compassion for this young man, she is brought face to face in the sharpest way with the inescapable implications of her own failing kidneys. This confrontation with the reality of her condition has, paradoxically, a sense of unreality about it. As Pat struggles to take in the implications of it all, it seems like 'this can't be happening'.

'Going back to that patient—I wonder was it best for him not to know that he was going into renal failure? Or should he have had five or six years of knowing and been prepared? There are two ways of looking at it; he had five years of peace and a sense of security, but then the shock. It's like when the doctor said to me I'd got five years before dialysis; when I started my dialysis within two years I felt cheated.'

As she witnessed the shock of the 'fit young man' and describes the shock of starting her own dialysis, the incomprehensible seems unreal. It is as if her nursing knowledge and her body collide. Her world, which had already been 'turned on its axis', is usurped by a new reality and is forever changed.

This stage of her story is profoundly a tale of being, in Frank's words,[4] 'shipwrecked by the storm of her disease' (p. 54) and the 'narrative wreckage' (p. 53) she experiences in the face of diagnosis and a disintegrating body: the stories she has in place, and by which she locates herself, are smashed and battered on the rocks of illness.

Interwoven with Pat's primary narrative—her illness story—are other stories: stories of friendship, of being a woman, of age and of motherhood. However, her telling of the illness story focused at this point primarily on its impact on her identity as a nurse. It seems important to maintain the place and priority of this here, since the form and way of telling signify both content and meaning. As Eisner[5] (p. 138–9) comments:

> There has been a growing realization in recent years among researchers of something that artists have long known in their bones; namely that form matters, that content and form cannot be separated, that how one says something is part and parcel of what is said.

AN ACTUAL VOCATION

'I've always wanted to be a nurse. I went to a spiritualist church and when I was about 17—my grandmother came through and she says, "You've always wanted to be a nurse." This medium didn't know who I was, and she said, "You used to bandage little dolls and put them in hospital". So I think it was an actual vocation. I suppose that was around the 70s. Also, I had quite a terrible childhood—so I wanted to escape home. So living-in meant I could escape … it was a way out into something that I wanted to do. I'd done work experience in a geriatric place; I got on well with all the staff and went back as a voluntary worker four years before I started my training.'

NURSE/PATIENT—PATIENT/NURSE

Pat found it very difficult to be positioned as a nurse *and* as a patient; the tension she experiences between these two ways of being and their polarised associations, feelings and thoughts points sharply to the difficulty in Western culture of being patient and healthcare professional at the same time. As Davies and Harré[6] note (p. 46):

> Once having taken up a particular position as one's own, a person inevitably sees the world from the vantage point of that position and in terms of the particular images, metaphors, story lines and concepts which are made relevant within the particular discursive practice in which they are positioned.

Although the concept of the 'wounded healer'[7,8] is well recognised, the power differential between the sick (patient) and the well (healer) is such that in practice it is very difficult to be both. This affected Pat's relationships with patients and also with her colleagues. Since Pat was a nurse before she was a patient–both in a temporal sense and also in the sense that this was the identity claim which took precedence for her—her nurse sense of self was most threatened *by* her renal failure, and her patient self was most threatening *to* her colleagues. The polarised positioning of medical practitioner and patient—which, as Bennet[9] notes, predominates in Western medicine, rests on the binary division of medical practitioner and patient. The implicit assumption of this duality is that a medical body is a healthy body, whereas a patient body is explicitly the sick body. She reflects on the implications of this:

'The people that you've worked with and joked with are looking down on you from a height—it's like they've become a different class and you've become a lower class,' she tells me.

I jump in—perhaps too readily—with the recognition of the loss of a sense of control that comes with illness, my empathy blurring with identification: 'So as a patient you're suddenly lower status … it's a loss of power in a sense, isn't it?'

'It *is*, and especially when you've been their colleague as well.'

And this shift back and forth between nurse and patient is ongoing and woven into the fabric of the day: 'Sometimes you went from being on duty straight into being a patient without any break in between', she tells me. 'I'd be on duty looking after patients, and they'd be setting my machine up ready for me.'

A KIND OF RAPE

Pat's experience of moving between the role of nurse, with responsibility and professional knowledge, and that of patient, whose responsibility is to be the passive recipient of care, is forcefully conveyed when she reflects on her relationship with the doctors, who were predominantly male.

'And with the doctors—some of them I'd flirted with, joked with, gone to parties with … and there they are looking at my chest, and it's difficult because you still see the man, and there he is as a doctor, and it's hard …'

'You feel exposed?' I ask.

'Yes, 'cos they're checking your heart and doing this and that and you feel sort of, not raped, but it is a kind of rape … it's like an exposure 'cos you know, everybody wears a hat and that's what they see when you're walking round briskly or whatever, or when you're at a party. But this—*this* is like a vulnerable state; you're in your nightie for a start.'

Her experience of colleagues having access to her body for medical procedures or nursing care left her with a sense that not only her professional mask but her social mask had been taken away. As Lawler writes, 'The body and sexuality are intimately interrelated but there are important differences between the sexes which are reflective of patriarchy'[10] (p. 112). Nettleton notes that medical examination can 'involve a level of intimacy that is not usual outside of a sexual encounter'[11] (p. 119). So, to be exposed in such a way by male doctors, who, according to the hierarchy of the institution and the gendered division of healthcare professions, are already in a more powerful position than a female nurse, is particularly difficult.

'It *is* a loss of power,' she emphasises.

'Yes, it's a very passive position to be in—you've lost that sense of control, that illusion of control that we think we have when we're well.' I am aware that my reflections are coming increasingly from my own frame of reference, and I wonder if this is appropriate, or helpful, or not. However, Pat then responds with a powerful analogy that conveys her own feeling:

'Yes, you *do*; you lose your self. I think it's like being stripped bare, and I don't mean clothes—I mean your soul in a way. Much later, when I lost my hair through treatment, it was like the final humiliation. Your hair was the last vestige of that modesty.'

Pat makes powerful use of Jungian archetypes to illustrate the polarities of patient and nurse. Earlier she had said, 'your persona changes' and here, she 'is stripped bare' to her 'soul'. The 'persona', according to Jung, is a mask that is designed to convey a particular impression, and to conceal the 'inner person' or 'soul'.[12,13] As her nurse 'persona' is taken from her, she loses the prestige it confers. She is no longer 'walking round briskly' but is 'in that bed'. In addition, when she loses her hair, her 'last vestige of modesty' has gone and she is 'stripped bare'.

'There's nothing there covering you; it's "here I am, naked." I thought they've seen everything, they've seen all my secrets, they've seen things that you wouldn't even tell your closest friend, but *they* have seen. And these people were friends, not in the intimate sense, but they were colleague-friends.'

As a female nurse whose diagnosis has snatched away her professional 'persona', she encounters the 'medical persona'[14] (p. 67) of the male doctors and feels 'naked'. Given that the majority of doctors and consultants are male, and the majority of nurses are female, the culture that Pat refers to as the 'hand-maiden scenario' means that the already existing power differentials are exacerbated in the most humiliating way.

Pat felt that she was no longer of 'equal standing'; while she knew that her work was 'exemplary', she felt she was no longer taken seriously as a nurse, and that she missed out on promotions for which she was eligible, 'because they knew that I would have to have time off sick. They didn't think I was up to the job and I suppose looking back on it perhaps I wasn't …'

THE BATTLE RAGES

As she looks back on this period, she comments, 'I think the worst thing I did was to have my treatment at the same place I worked; I should've moved elsewhere.' In the unique position of being a nurse and a patient on the same ward, she reflects; 'You see things in different lights—you know. You look at the way nurses treat the patients, and you think that's not right—not that they were being cruel, but at times there is a lack of understanding. I've done it myself—when you're tired, you can be a bit short and you don't think anything of it. But when you're on the receiving end and you're feeling vulnerable and needy, sometimes you want the responsibility of the day taken off you. I can understand why patients become helpless in a way because they want that load lifted; it's too much for them to bear each day.'

She steps back into her nurse's shoes and the 'day-to-day reality of it', and comments:

'But you've got a job to do, and a limited amount of time to spend with each patient. So that's *the battle which rages inside you*—because you can see the nurses' point of view, and you can see the patients' and I tend to defend the nurses because that's where I'm coming from; I'm not the patient, I am the nurse. It's very hard to reconcile the two.'

Her colleagues reacted in different and sometimes unexpected ways: 'Some were very supportive and kind, but others were very dismissive. They wouldn't give that little bit of leeway … I felt like they thought less of me because of my illness.'

The sharp ambiguity of her position cuts deep for Pat, and also for some of her colleagues. She told of an occasion when someone had suggested she write something for a nursing journal from a patient-nurse point of view: 'I mentioned it to the transplant coordinator and he said, "Oh well, they'll just say that you've jumped on the bandwagon, that because of your experience you want something published", and that "it would be seen as capitalising".'

She felt that the suggestion was seen as inappropriate, and thus she was denied access to a context in which she might have had a voice.

'If I had said I wanted to write an article before I became a patient, he would have accepted it. But it was like, "you can't use your misfortune to gain". But I wasn't looking at it that way; it was just an idea I was kicking around which someone had mentioned. And I thought it would be good for people to know what it was like.'

The incident somehow crystallises the difficulty and the subtleties of being in both worlds, where her positioning as a patient meant that she was effectively denied access to a domain of language use preserved for nurses. According to Foucault, the discourses to which we have access 'are the bearers of the specific effects of power'[15] (p. 94): the inseparability of knowledge and power meant that, as a patient, Pat's professional voice was suspect and silenced. As White and Epston[16] (p. 22) put it:

> Since we are all caught up in a net or web of power/knowledge, it is not possible to act apart from this domain, and we are simultaneously undergoing the effects of power and exercising this power in relation to others.

'So once you were in the situation of being on dialysis, even though you were still working as a nurse, it felt as though your professional status was being wrenched away from you?' I ask.

'Yes, and perhaps my own confidence was eroded; you do lose a lot of your authority as well, and you doubt your own ability 'cos people are doubting you. I think it's an erosion that happens from the moment you are diagnosed and you don't realise it.'

The complexity and ambiguity of power are brought sharply into focus by serious illness. Pat's experience of a shift in power in relation to her professional status highlights the fragility of such status. She recognises how complex this is for her colleagues: 'It's difficult for them as well; they still treat you as their colleague in a way, because they'll tell you things … but I felt like I'd been demoted.'

One of the effects of Pat's ambiguous status is that the particular and special insight that she offered as both nurse and patient was overlooked. Yet as Kapur, in the preface to a collection of first-person accounts written by clinicians who have sustained brain injury, comments: 'Doctors and other clinicians who become patients provide a unique perspective of the healer who now needs to be healed'[17] (p. vii).

It was almost as if by becoming a patient as well as a nurse, she had not only blurred the boundaries, but she had transgressed, and 'gone over to the other side'. Bennet views the 'denial of death' as one of the main defensive attitudes by which doctors may maintain a sense of power and control. He writes, 'If doctors have profound anxieties about their own mortality, they will become uncomfortable when facing it in a patient. If the patient is one of them, mortality comes that much closer'[18] (p. 82). As practitioners, part of their sense of agency and identity would have resided in the 'restitution narrative'[19] (p. 75) in which their primary role is to restore health; somehow when 'one of their own' was under threat, it was also a threat to their own professional identities.

'Sick colleagues,' according to Bennet, 'present the greatest emotional challenges to doctors'[20] (p. 84). As Pat expresses it, 'Looking back on my relationships with some of the people at work, perhaps they couldn't cope with my illness; it was too difficult.'

DEALING WITH LIFE AND DEATH

'And at work you can't wear your heart on your sleeve all the time because you couldn't cope. When I first started nursing, I used to come home, and if it had been quite a traumatic time, I just used to sit and I couldn't speak to anyone for an hour or so. It's one of the reasons why I started smoking. A lot of nurses smoke as a way of coping, and especially when we were training. Nurses have a reputation of being a bit wild … because you have to, you have to. But I think it's a way of unwinding, of saying that you're alive or something. With nursing—because you are dealing with life and death—you can't help but become fond of people and have feelings for the family … because it's a very emotional time and bonds are formed very quickly. And although that patient is there for three or four weeks or longer, you can get a lifetime of living in that time because you are laid bare; there's no reason to put on airs and graces.'

I say, 'I find that really moving, Pat: your sense of connection with people. You are living, and you are sharing people's mortality. You're right in there—it's human life at its most extreme.'

'It's raw … raw. When I was on the wards and they did die, it was the last rites … the last thing anybody's going to do for this person; you feel such respect and it's such a privilege to do that for them.

'But', she observes, 'some people can't handle illnesses—they can't. And they walk away. Perhaps my colleagues couldn't handle it so close to home.'

It is almost as if Pat's colleagues felt that if she, a nurse on a dialysis unit, could have renal failure, then so could they. The next time we meet, Pat tells me of a recent conversation with one of her former colleagues.

'We were discussing my experiences when I was dialysed and working there. Like I told you, some people weren't very supportive, but on reflection perhaps they couldn't cope. She (my colleague) said, "It was like we were all play acting, it was so surreal to have to look after you—not that I didn't want to … but to do the things that we were doing for the patients to one of our own." She said, "It was quite difficult putting tubes down your nose like we used to do in training."'

'It's almost like there's a divide between healthcare professionals on the one side and patients on the other, isn't it, and you'd kind of crossed over,' I suggest.

'Yeah, sort of straddling it,' Pat responds, picking up and extending the metaphor. 'We were talking about mortality, and I told her how I felt about it, and she said, "I can't identify with you because I have never experienced my mortality and therefore I've still got the luxury of not knowing". And for her to articulate it like that brought it home to me how people actually feel … and because it's been so long since I felt safe myself … I felt envious, actually. But at the time when I was in it, I was supported by a fair number of people, and without them, I don't think I would have got through. I really don't, and I will be grateful for that,' she adds.

RELATIONSHIPS WITH PATIENTS

Pat's diagnosis and treatment also affected her relationships with patients. She felt that being treated in the unit where she worked took away her privacy and choice about this; 'I didn't want what was private to become public knowledge. I felt for it to be common knowledge compromised my position as a nurse. I'd think, well you know, I'm here to look after you. And of course people react differently. Some patients were really supportive, and they'd say, "Well you know what it means and how it goes," and, I'd say, "Well yes I do, I know exactly where you're coming from." But other patients would say, "Well it's all right for you, you're a nurse, so you know about it"; as if you could actually govern how you were feeling, how your illness progressed!'

A WAITING GAME

In a written account of the issues relating to renal failure, Pat observes, 'There is never an acceptance of life on dialysis, and hope is focussed on being successfully transplanted. There is a sense of suspension from life, even if day-to-day living seems normal. To be faced with a future, watching what you eat, only allowed 500–750 mls of fluid daily and dependent on a machine is demoralising. A transplant is a dream, hearing about other patients who we transplant, there is naturally a tinge of envy amid the celebrations.'

'When they said about home dialysis, we moved here and they put that extension on for us, and that's where I used to have my dialysis. But I don't really like the room anymore … I very rarely … it's just a junk room … if I had my own way, I would have it taken down …

'I just got on with dialysis as best you can,' she continues. 'Lots of other people were being transplanted, and sometimes I would catch myself wishing it was me. You feel happy for that person but you can't help feel a bit envious … it's a human thing. So I just waited; it was a waiting game. I didn't panic every time the phone rang. I thought, when it happens, it happens. It does get you down though. You've got to plan your nights out, watch what you eat and drink. It never leaves your brain. It's always there. It affects your relationship with your partner; obviously the physical side deteriorates because you don't have the libido; and also your relationship with your children 'cos you're tired and everything revolves round you, and they get neglected. So they're living it with you, and they don't see you the same.'

The next time we meet, I say, 'I guess this is stirring up quite a lot for you …'

'It is,' she nods. 'As I'm talking to you, I'm reliving some of it in my head. I'm telling you bits of it, but in my mind I can see the whole scenario playing out … and the emotions. I'm telling you part of it, but in my mind the rest of it is happening.'

I think of stories that go untold for all sorts of reasons: because they are paradoxical, or contradictory; because of dominant discourses, because they are just too painful to tell or to hear; or because experience may be too complex and chaotic for linear stories.

Pat talks of the death of Caroline, her closest friend. 'She was such an honest person, and she wasn't scared of talking about her feelings. She was a nurse herself, and she was quite open with me in every aspect of her illness. And I felt privileged, you know, because they were private thoughts … When she died, it changed me. Prior to that, I didn't like to upset people. I was quite timid really. But afterwards, you look at things and think, "Well the little things are not important". It was such a profound time in my life. And if she had been alive, the whole thing would have been different,' she reflects.

TRANSPLANT

I ask Pat about her transplant: 'So can you tell me how that happened?'

'Well I was on dialysis for nearly two years. And then one morning, I was getting ready for work. It was about 5 o'clock, and I got that phone call. I was so calm. John was in a panic, but I was so calm. She said, "This is the transplant co-ordinator; just sit down and do this." She told me exactly what to do. She was so calm, and it helped a lot; she gave me a list of things to do. So I got on the machine and dialysed, and we talked for about two hours while I was on. She was married to someone on dialysis, and he was transplanted, so she knew from both sides herself.

'John was in such a panic, and I said, "Oh we'll just pop to the shops—I want to get some new nighties." "Shopping!" John says. "Well I've got to get them," I told him. "I want some nice stuff, toiletries and things." When we got to the hospital, there was an air of excitement. Then I had a phone call from the surgeon, and he said, "I can't do your operation—I'm running a bit late because I'm doing this child. So it'll be later on".

'I was just thinking about this 2-year-old child, and then someone told me that the transplant came from a 19-year-old boy; he'd been in a car crash that morning. Well the floodgates just opened. I was so upset ... I kept thinking those parents have experienced such loss—I was thinking to myself how I would feel—and they had the *kindness* to give to me. I was so humbled; it's such a humbling experience, you know, to think of someone's thoughts—and yet they said yes. And it's such a responsibility; it *feels* like a responsibility 'cos you take on board all that emotion. And I was in tears and I kept thinking of this little baby at the children's hospital and they were saying the surgeon was having difficulty getting the kidney connected, 'cos he was so tiny. Then he eventually rang about eight, and he said, "I'm too tired to do your kidney operation today; I'll do it in the morning, first thing." He was very hands-on. And I was thinking of this young man going out for the evening, and this little baby, so tiny. I was in tears.

'I was transplanted in the morning, and afterwards it didn't take very well. That was a bad time; the kidney went to sleep. It wouldn't work and I had to have dialysis. Sometimes the shock of being taken out and put into the recipient means it goes to sleep. Obviously I was on the transplant ward and all these patients were coming in during the night and they were peeing buckets—they had catheters full! And I used to go, "There, look! That's what you're supposed to be doing!"' she laughs. 'But it did start to work ... you just had to keep drinking loads to try and encourage it. And then when it started it wouldn't stop!'

HEART ATTACK

'I came home two days before Christmas, and I was rushing round Tesco's and started to feel really breathless. I had this pain here.' She points to her chest. 'And it was getting quite bad. And this had also happened before I was discharged; during my recovery I was getting all this pain—they put me on the ECG monitor and just put it down to stress. It was so frightening; I just wanted someone to sit with me, and I knew that they couldn't because they were busy. I used to phone John, and he used to come and sleep the night beside my bed.

'So on New Year's Eve—millennium eve—I was getting all this indigestion and pain, and so I went upstairs. I thought I'll just have five minutes; and it just felt like terrible, terrible indigestion. About 11 o'clock I said, "You'll have to phone for an ambulance". I was having a heart attack. Your mind becomes quite surreal at the time, because although it's happening to you, you're not scared; you get anaesthetised. I don't remember feeling frightened … they had to rush me to hospital. I had to have an angiogram and it showed a blockage and it was angina; and so I felt quite betrayed at that stage 'cos I'd spoken to my GP and to my renal consultant, and everyone said, oh it's a bit of asthma. They hadn't taken me seriously.

'And then my kidney started failing. At times, I really wished I hadn't been transplanted 'cos I didn't have these problems. I put on loads of weight because of all the steroids. Then I lost all my hair and all the weight; I was so thin, at one stage they were thinking of drip feeding me. Nobody told me that I was going to be so ill, and that was a shock. Because my immune system was so low, I was full of cold sores and ulcers. The flesh was just hanging because the weight was lost so quickly. I was in a dreadful state.'

Transplant is commonly seen as a means of 'restitution': as the cure which restores normality. The 'restitution narrative'[21] (p. 75), which prevails in contemporary Western societies, views the body as 'a kind of car' which 'breaks down and has to be repaired' (p. 86). It is, as Frank puts it, an attempt to 'outdistance mortality by rendering illness transitory'[22] (p. 115). The discourse of restitution exerts a cultural pressure to return to the person you were before the illness. However, renal failure is a chronic, long-term condition and transplant is, in effect, a means of management rather than of cure. Therefore a sense of uncertainty and of ongoing disruption continues: as Pat has written, 'although transplanted and free from dialysis, it feels transient'. With ongoing illness, such as renal failure, Pat is not only dealing with temporary interruption but with 'perpetual vulnerability to interruption' in which 'tidy ends are no longer appropriate to the story'[23] (p. 59).

50:50

Pat's heart and renal problems persisted over the next few months. When I next see her, she takes up the story from where she left off:

'I had a line in my neck for dialysis, and they were using it for drugs, and also for taking blood because my veins weren't very good. So they left it in. I had angina, and in June they said I needed a heart bypass. I was getting quite ill—I had septicaemia through this line, so they tried to take it out. But they couldn't—it was wedged right into my ventricle, so they were pulling it; these are all the scars. I was really quite ill; they were consulting all sorts of people to try and bring my infection down. It was a terrible time; I was in a terrible state.

'In August, they tried three times to take me to theatre to take the line out and to have a bypass. But each time they had to cancel 'cos of my temperature. In the end, the surgeon came to me … he said, "I'll lay it on the line; you've got a 50:50 chance, because you might make it and you might not. It's quite serious this time, and I've got to do it to give you any chance. I'm going to try and do the bypass at the same time if I can—but I think we'll have to replace the valve because there's growth there." That's when it really hit me that I could die. And the shock of it—I dunno … you look at things and everything seems brighter and sounds seem louder. Everything was heightened … and I didn't say anything to him 'cos I couldn't.

'The morning of my heart operation, they came for me very early. I was quite calm in a way. When you're faced like that—I dunno about you—but I'd made my peace … with the world … or whichever god you believe in. You *are* at peace, aren't you?'

'Yeah,' I respond. 'I remember seeing other patients wheeled down to theatre and thinking one day that will be me. And how am I gonna feel? And when it was me, I was as ready to face that as I've ever been to face anything in my life.'

'I knew that I might not be coming back, but I just felt I'd be with Caroline, that there would be someone there for me,' she says.

'And so you had a sense of connection with her? A sense that you were close to her, whatever…whether you came through or you didn't. Is that right?' I ask.

'Yes, 'cos it took the fear away—it just took the fear away.'

But, as Barone writes, 'Good stories rattle commonplace assumptions and disturb taken-for-granted beliefs'[24] (p. 223). At the same time as telling the story of preparing herself for the possibility of dying, Pat also tells an alternative story, and offers a counterplot.

'And then when I woke up, I was quite angry! 'Cos I felt cheated!' She roars with laughter.

Laughing, I say, 'Almost like you'd prepared yourself for one thing!'

'Yeah—it was like a rebirth! It was such a shock!' She laughs.

'So you woke up … and you were almost shocked to be still here?'

'Yeah—it's all over and you don't expect to be alive!'

'You wake up and you are alive … thinking what's going on here!' I respond.

'Yeah … what's this!? And then as soon as I was awake, I was awake! I remember feeling very uncomfortable with the intubating tube. And I couldn't move very well. And I remember, my hand was here, and I got to the end. And the nurse thought, "She's gonna pull her tube out!" And it was down again! John said, "I knew you were going to be all right, 'cos you were being naughty again!"' She roars with laughter.

'You know the probe they put on your finger—the oxygen thing,' I say. 'I remember playing and flicking it off. And it stopped beeping. And I got told off. So I did it again! It was just that little …'

'Devilment …' she affirms.

'Mischief …' I say.

'Reasserting yourself!' she responds.

There is a fundamental paradox in 'living with mortality'; on the one hand, Pat is preparing herself for death, and on the other, she shows vitality and humour when her preparations are thwarted.

Pat's operation was successful, and she made a gradual recovery. However, the long-term nature of her condition is such that she will always have to be monitored.

A transplanted kidney has a limited 'life span', and therefore she continues to live with uncertainty, and a sense that she can never take her life for granted.

Tentatively, I say, 'A couple of weeks back you said I'll be lucky if I get to 50, and I wondered how you feel about that and how you see it? You've mentioned it a couple of times. And I've said similar; it's something I've done too; it's how it is to live with a heightened sense of your own mortality, isn't it?'

'It *is*—you are aware of it; you've been to the brink and you know it's there. It *is* your mortality. You've hit the nail on the head. It's like having a death sentence, but you don't know when the execution day will be. And I get really panicky … John has never had anything wrong with him—his mam's 93, and he doesn't see. I see death more clearly than he does; he'll take things for granted and I can't, because I don't have that luxury anymore.'

'Yes,' I reply, 'and it *is* a luxury, isn't it; you can't take it for granted—not anymore.'

'You can't; death is a fact of life,' she says.

'Yes, it *is* a fact of life; there's no getting away from it, is there? I don't know if this rings any bells for you but I remember, in the days leading up to my own surgery, looking at my children and knowing that there was quite a strong chance that I wouldn't see them grow up, and that was the most indescribably painful thing. And you presumably had similar moments …'

Both slightly tearful. 'I think it's, erm …' She swallowed. 'It's, erm, leaving them behind, actually … my son only visited me a couple of times in hospital, and I thought he didn't care … and afterwards he said to me, "I couldn't bear it, mam …"'

'As you were talking,' I say, 'I remember a time when things looked pretty grim and it did look like I might well not … and my son couldn't look at me; I could see the pain on his face and I remember feeling so helpless. I wanted to take that pain away and I couldn't—and he just knew; it was one of the saddest things I've ever experienced in my life.'

'Yeah' …' she pauses; 'That's when you think there's no one for him to go to. It's like when you're driving along and you think, oh god, if we had an accident, he'd be on his own …'

There is stillness in the room. Traffic hums in the distance, but in here, there is sadness you could touch.

CHAINS THAT PIN AND BIND

She talks of the changes that illness has brought:

'I mean, you just get on with it, don't you, you have to … but when you look back … sometimes it's too much … I mean—like with dialysis—you dream of simple things, like coffee, or tomato soup … just silly things. There have always been restraints throughout my life; if it's not dietary, it's something, and that idealistic person gets knocked out; a chain thrown here, a chain thrown there, and if it's not racism, it's sexism; they're all chains, and they pin you and bind you. So you can't be a butterfly and flutter here and there.'

She pauses, 'When I was nursing—on a geriatric ward—this old lady had died, and they found a poem in her locker. The gist of it was: "You've seen me here, all wrinkled and old, but do you know my hopes and my dreams when I was young?" The world sees her as a little old lady, but inside she's still that vital woman.'

I think of her words when I last saw her; she said: 'It's changed me; I look at my body—it makes you less of a woman, you know. I'd been quite a feminine woman. I liked my high heels, my stockings … but I can't wear them anymore. You look at yourself and you think, there's a big blob in the mirror.'

And I say, 'That's the sense that I get of you; that you feel that your body has changed on the outside, but inside you're still that vital woman. It's funny, but when I was driving here, I was listening to a Neil Young song, and it's a story about this girl who rides a Harley Davidson and she rides off into the sunset with her hair flying in the wind … so when you said that, the song just came into my mind …'

She nods. 'Yes. You know, I was thinking—we're going to a party next week, and I thought, why can't I wear my high heels? So I went out and bought a really high pair of sexy shoes!'

She laughs uproariously—and so do I. 'Oh, wow, fantastic!' I exclaim.

'I thought, well, I'll wear them and if my feet start swelling up, I'll have another pair in the car—because you make too many excuses, don't you? I thought, I'm just gonna walk in there, in me shoes.

'I mean there's a friend of mine, and he has a sports car, and the car represents who he is,' she says.

I wonder, 'What do you think would represent you?'

'A big walrus at the moment,' she laughs.

'And the butterfly?' I ask. 'The you that wants to fly?'

'Well … yes … I mean, like these shoes ... yeah, they're ridiculous! And I think, that *is* me. It's just that sometimes you want to *be* that person, don't you? You want to *be* who you are inside; you want to *be* that outside, as well. And I can't get into the clothes that I'd really like to wear, but I *can* get into these shoes … it's just a little bit of rebellion, I suppose …'

She pauses, 'Like my friend; we went to a tattoo parlour not so long ago. I had a fantastic time in there. I was enthralled … the blokes were like ZZ Top; biker blokes. They looked so fierce, and they were really nice … it's like they represented freedom; on their bikes, doing what they wanted. She's 57, my friend, and she had a little devil put on her shoulder … I suppose it's an expression of yourself … she sees herself as a little devil … and she's bigger than I am. But she's still got that rebellion in her.'

'And you have it in you, haven't you?' I venture.

'So have you!' she counters. She roars with laughter, and I do too.

As I pack away my tapes and prepare to leave, Patricia says, 'Just a minute', and goes upstairs. She returns with a pair of shoes: red suede, elegant and vital.

'Look, they've got 3½inch heels!' she exclaims.

'Oh wow—they're gorgeous! And very sexy!'

As I drive home, I wonder about meaning, purpose and identity. I wonder about the ethics of finding my own meaning and purpose in researching and writing about the illness experience of others. For I know that my movement into writing and research is rooted in my own loss, and that my work has been a site for developing a new voice and a new sense of self. I accelerate onto the motorway. As I join the traffic streaming south, the 'Angel of the North' watches over. Neil Young sings, 'She gets the faraway look in her eyes'.[25] I think of beautiful shoes and my saxophone in its case under my bed. It lies there, its golden sound unvoiced; for now that I can no longer play it, I can hardly bear to look at it.

REFERENCES

1   Aristotle. *Poetics*. Heath M, translator. London: Penguin; 1996

2. Bruner J. *Making Stories: law, literature, life*. New York: Farrar, Straus and Giroux; 2002: pp. 4–6.

3. Bruner J. *Actual Minds, Possible Worlds*. Cambridge, MA: Harvard University Press; 1986.

4. Frank A. *The Wounded Storyteller: body, illness and ethics*. Chicago, IL: University of Chicago Press; 1995.

5. Eisner EW. Concerns and aspirations for qualitative research in the new millennium. *Qual Res*. 2001; **1**(2): 135–45.

6. Davies B, Harré R. Positioning: the discursive production of selves. *J Theory Soc Behav*. 1990; **20**: 4–63.

7. Jung CG. *The Practice of Psychotherapy. (Vol. 16, The Collected Works.)* London: Routledge and Kegan Paul; 1954.

8. Nouwen HJM. *The Wounded Healer: ministry in contemporary society*. New York, NY: Image Books; 1990.

9. Bennet G. *The Wound and the Doctor: healing, technology and power in modern medicine*. London: Secker and Warburg; 1987.

10. Lawler J. *Behind the Screens: nursing, somology and the problem of the body*. London: Churchill Livingstone; 1991.

11. Nettleton S. *The Sociology of Health and Illness*. London: Polity Press; 1995.

12. Jung CG. *Two Essays on Analytical Psychology. (Vol. 7, The Collected Works.)* London: Routledge and Kegan Paul; 1953.

13. Jung CG. *Selected Writings*. In: Storr A, editor. London: Fontana; 1983.

14. Nouwen, op cit.

15. Foucault M. *Power/Knowledge: Selected interviews and other writings*. Gordon C, editor. New York: Pantheon Books; 1980.

16. White M, Epston D. *Narrative Means to Therapeutic Ends*. New York: Norton; 1990.

17. Kapur N. *Injured Brains of Medical Minds*. New York, NY: Oxford University Press; 1997.

18. Bennet, op cit.
19. Frank, op.cit.
20. Bennet, op cit.
21. Frank, op cit.
22. Frank, op cit.
23. Bruner, 1986, op cit.
24. Barone T. Among the chosen: a collaborative educational (auto)biography. *Qualitative Inquiry.* 1997; **3**(2): 222–36.
25. Young N. Unknown Legend. *Harvest Moon* [recording]. Reprise; 1992.

CHAPTER 3

Jan's story

INTRODUCTION

Jan is in her mid-20s and was born with a congenital hip dislocation. This means that she spent considerable time in hospital as a child, and also as a teenager having orthopaedic surgery. It also means that she lives with hip problems and the prospect of further surgery at some stage in her life. She is a psychologist and at the time of these conversations was engaged in her own PhD research.

The hip is a joint which consists of a ball (the end of the leg bone) and a cup-shaped socket in the hip bone. All newborn babies have their hips checked for instability in this joint, since dislocation, if not detected and treated early, can lead to long-term problems, pain and reduced mobility from arthritis or further damage to the joint. Treatment can involve traction, splinting, plaster cast or surgery. Jan's hip difficulties were not detected until she started to walk, and she has needed operations on her hips at different points throughout her life.

Jan and I had met previously in a work context, and she knew I was a counsellor and teacher. She also knew that I had been ill and had written about it. When I contacted her to enquire whether she would be interested in participating, she told me that she felt it would be beneficial to her in developing 'personal insight' into the relationship between her experience and her identity.

After contact through phone and email, we met to talk through the ethical issues and practicalities. I began by asking Jan, 'If you had never met me, and you wanted to tell me about that experience in your childhood, how would you start?'

I'D PROBABLY START WITH THE FACTS

'I think I'd probably start with the facts, to be honest … but saying that now, I've realised that I don't really know the facts, because I was so young at the time. I couldn't go through and say, in this year I had this operation or that operation; obviously I don't remember. Both hips were dislocated when I was born, but they didn't pick it up till I started walking. I went into the orthopaedic hospital when I was two apparently for about a year on and off.'

Research into memory in recent years suggests that memory is constructed as well as stored.[1,2] As Jan considers 'the facts', she goes on to explore and construct memories which convey a 'narrative truth'[3] that adequately captures her experience. Spence[4] defines 'narrative truth' as 'the criterion we use to decide when a certain experience has been captured to our satisfaction; it depends on continuity and closure and the extent to which the fit of the pieces (of the story) takes on an aesthetic finality' (p. 31). Jan goes on to retrace sensory impressions and puts these together with other sources of information, such as family stories. In doing so, she creates a narrative truth that is meaningful and 'fits' the 'pieces' of her story. This accommodates her 'felt-sense'[5] and 'tacit knowledge'[6,7] of these early experiences, and represents her embodied perceptions. Indeed, Rosenfield[8] emphasises the idea that 'recollection is a kind of perception … and every context will alter the nature of what is recalled' (p. 89). Our memories are individual perceptions that are embodied and informed by our personal, social and cultural histories. Our use of language enables us to move beyond bodily awareness of sensation and emotion, and to create more explicit and coherent memories through narrative, and with regard to context. Jan later refers to our meetings as an opportunity to tell a 'joined up, flowing story' as opposed to occasions such as the medical context when 'I might tell bits of it, but probably not so much the emotional side of things'. As Etherington[9] writes, 'When we accept that memory is not necessarily something concrete that needs to be 'unearthed', but rather a 'gathering together' of different kinds of information, images, metaphors and responses, we become free to explore creatively, flexibly and spontaneously …' (p. 53). As Jan 'gathers together' these different sources of information, she creates and constructs her early memories. It is this creative capacity of memory that enables us to process and transform traumatic experience, in ways which can be healing. I have chosen to represent Jan's 'first memories' in stanza form since I feel it evokes their sensory impressionistic nature more effectively:[10,11,12]

First memories
Hospital …
That's where my first memories are …
I suppose that's linked to the experience
'Cos it's a different experience
Not the usual memories …
But things like … quite sensory things
The smell and
The sound and
The sights

Being wheeled down to the operating theatre
And the gas mask…..
The scariest feeling
Like you were being smothered

I remember when I was first in
when I was very little
looking out through the window
for mum
coming in every day

I always remember that

I remember when I was two and a half
my dad
coming in every night

He would read me Peter Rabbit
And I knew the words
I'd remember if he missed out a word
I suppose the memories I have relate really to family

Bateson[13] writes, 'Human sense organs can receive *only* news of difference and the differences must be coded into events in time' (p. 79). Jan's earliest associations are the smells, the sounds and the sights of hospital—'not the usual memories' but 'a different experience', which is embodied. As she remembers her dad reading to her, she signals the immediacy of her experiential memory by moving imperceptibly into the historic present tense:

Looking out of the window
I can just picture it now
Seeing my mum
oh everything's going to be alright now

The poignancy of her sensory memories take us into the experience of the little girl looking out for her mum, and vividly show how our senses receive this 'news of difference', which is later 'coded into events in time'. As Jan looks back on her infancy, she notes that these sensory impressions signal the unanticipated, highlighting Bruner's[14] observation that both as children and adults we 'are highly attuned to the unexpected' (p. 31).

AMBIVALENCE

Jan spent a lot of time in hospital throughout her childhood and adolescence, and therefore it was an environment with particularly powerful associations and complex meanings.

'The feelings it evokes are quite strong, actually. If I drive past the orthopaedic hospital—it's strange—there's a sense of nervousness but a sense of belonging as well.'

'A sense of connection?' I ask.

'Yeah—that's really quite strong. And when I was younger, it was a familiar place, but yesterday I realised that I was going close to it and I thought, Oh …' She shivers. 'And I didn't actually go past it in the end, but it was that sense of, Oh god, I'm gonna go past it …'

Because these are such experiential sensory memories, it seems to me that it is important to stay with them at this stage. Jan's early memories convey a powerful sense of her early childhood experience and tell us something about the hospital environment and the complex feelings it can generate. This was particularly pertinent for her at the time of our conversations, as she was starting to experience pain in her hips once again. Therefore my questions, within the 'landscape of consciousness', focus on exploring these associations and meanings.[15,16,17]

'It's strange 'cos I don't ever think back to when I was in hospital and my operations with a sense of being scared. But I suppose it's the feeling of not wanting to get back into that.'

The hospital experience can generate deeply ambivalent feelings for any of us. But for a child to be separated from her parents it can be particularly difficult. The work of Bowlby[18,19] on attachment and separation was starting to influence the development of policies on 'open' visiting for children in hospital but this was still in its early stages.[20,21,22] As Jan observes, at that time—the mid-1970s—'mums weren't allowed to stay', and she has abiding memories of 'looking out for mum through the window'. Security and safety coexist for her alongside uncertainty and fear. There is a sense of belonging and community alongside separation and isolation:

'Hospital was always quite a safe environment, despite the surgery. I remember it as not being a particularly difficult time—although, obviously, the first night and mum going … But after that, it was nice; I have fond memories.'

'So you formed quite strong attachments and connections with the place and people?' I ask.

'Yes, very much so; I remember going back when I was a bit older and looking onto the ward and thinking fond memories. I had a sense of attachment and bonding to the people there because there was a kind of sameness with the other children; you weren't different,' she observes. 'I remember it as quite a safe, familiar time. But ...' she reflects, 'if I think about going back for an MRI, there is some fear to it as well, isn't there?' Her question tag denotes recognition of shared experience. 'Some anxiety … the smell … and nothing ever changes. It's an old hospital … and everything's always the same … only smaller and more intense.'

The hospital that figured large in her childhood seems 'smaller' when she is older, but also 'more intense' in what it represents. The smell and the fact that 'nothing ever changes' gives Jan a sense of anxiety and fear. Smell, in evolutionary terms, is one of the oldest parts of our brains and is associated with emotion, and with the fight or flight response; this connection with survival is one of the reasons why smell can evoke memories so strongly. As Alaoui-Ismaïli[23] states, 'complex and numerous central olfactory projections link to structures in the limbic system, in particular amygdala and hippocampus, implicated in the modulation of emotion' (p. 238).

Jan recalls going to the hospital for a magnetic resonance imaging (MRI) scan and looking in on the children's ward, which is next to the radiology department:

> As you went in, there was a little gate
> And then a corridor with rooms off it
> there was the first bay and the second bay,
> then the nurses station,
> the third bay and the fourth bay for the older children
>
> And I remember thinking
> I've worked my way through each these bays, as I've grown up
> And it's such a big part of my upbringing …
>
> My first memories are before they built the children's ward
> We were in a kind of shack in the grounds
> And at one end they had a curtained off area
> where they'd take your stitches out
>
> And I remember being really fearful of the curtain …
> Scary …

I think of my own associations … when I go for MRI scans and how these always take me—whoosh—straight back into not just factual memories but the immediacy of my first scans. For Jan, these associations are woven into the fabric of her growing up, and her images of 'the shack' and 'the curtain' evoke an almost tangible sense of the fear relating to procedures such as when 'they'd take your stitches out'.

RELATIONSHIPS

As a child spending so much time in hospital, the relationships within that environment are fundamentally important; she valued the sense of 'sameness' with the other children, and had talked of 'attachment and bonding'. I ask her what she remembers about the staff.

'The nurses were just an absolute lifeline—they were fantastic—they were so caring and very different to the doctors. Certainly, as a child, I thought the doctors were there to do their job. They'd come round and stand at the end of your bed and talk about you without you being there. I don't even feel—well obviously, I do have a sense of gratitude to them—but I was always so much more grateful to the nurses, who'd given the time and got to know you; but the medics … they were highly skilled and highly trained, and they do their job … It was quite interesting that when parents came in, they didn't just talk to their own child but there was a sense of, "Can I get you something?" and of everybody in there together,' she says.

'A kind of community?' I ask.

'Yes, and a very caring community,' she adds. 'And I remember one thing that always kept us going on the ward—everybody loved it: there was one cleaner who was the spitting image of Yazz. Do you remember that song of hers, "The Only Way is Up"?'

'Oh yes, I do,' I say.

'Well, she was so funny—she used to make everybody's day. She'd be saying, "What's the matter with you, pull yourself together!" But mixed in with humour, and it was such a good way of helping us in getting on with things and getting through the day. And in a sense, we needed that, 'cos so many had just had operations. And I remember the school; the teacher was great, and she kept us going as well.'

Jan's repeated periods in hospital are set against the backdrop of an English education system, where at eleven or twelve, the transition from primary school to secondary school takes place. This transition coincided with one of Jan's operations.

A SENSE OF DIFFERENCE

'When I started secondary school, I was late because it coincided with my operation when I was 12. Everybody else had started and I was going into the unknown, into a much bigger school.'

> I remember going back to school afterwards
> I was on crutches,
> and that sense of …
> aloneness
> of difference
> of being more vulnerable
>
> At home there was always mum and dad and my sister
> Doing more or less the same jobs as the nurses
>
> So to go back to school …
> It felt like I'd had my cotton wool ripped off from around me.
> You become more lost in the crowd
>
> When you're in hospital
> You've been looked after
> People are looking out for you
> Whereas that's gone at school
>
> And there was that sense of difference
> I had to use the lift at school
> (which everybody else wanted to use too!)
> It was having to start late
> Then being different as well

As Becker[24] writes, 'Stories of disruption are, by definition, stories of difference. Disruption makes an individual feel different from others' (p. 16). Jan reflects on the nature of this difference:

'In a way, a lot of my childhood was around my hips and what that brought with it. I suppose, as a child, there was a kind of specialness about me because of it. I do remember when I was first in, as a two year old, and as a child, it kind of brought the family system together. Mum would be in every day, dad would come in, and then there was my sister, who must have felt very left out. And my grandparents came in. So I had that sense of being quite central to the family process when I was in hospital. And then through school—even though I didn't like having the scars—there were always people interested. But there *was* that sense of being a bit different, and at that stage, it wasn't a difference that I was very uncomfortable with. It was going through adolescence that I started to feel *more* uncomfortable about being "different"'.

We have a sense of what is the 'normal' social order according to our gender, age, social class and particular circumstances. Deeply embedded discourses on the family, on education and on career choices inform expectations, hopes and fears. As Becker[25] points out, 'they are all moral discourses' which 'reflect dominant ideologies about how life should be lived' (p. 16). Feeling different from others is fundamental for Jan since her condition is 'inherent to being me'. Jan doesn't face the disruption of sudden acute illness but has had a sense of being different and of being vulnerable to disruption throughout her life.

I ask her how going into hospital in her teens felt compared to her experiences as a child.

'I was getting to a stage when I didn't want it to be so much a part of my life, and it felt like it was disrupting everything and getting in the way. It felt more serious, and I felt more alone, even though I wasn't. I just had that sense of being on my own and dealing with it on my own much more than when I was younger.'

'You said it felt more serious—in what sense did it feel more serious?'

'I think because it was interrupting my life. School was disrupted; I was getting into my GCSE year. It was really interfering with friendships. And I just didn't want a whole summer holiday in hospital. And it was encroaching onto term time as well. I wanted to be like everybody else without this. And I was the oldest on the ward then, so there was that sense of having outgrown this. I didn't want to belong to it as well. But I *did* belong to it …' she tails off.

This most difficult sense of belonging, a belonging to a community that she has 'outgrown', separates Jan from her teenage life and seems to me to be such a lonely kind of belonging. I ask her about this.

'When you talk about when you were a small child there was a sense of not being alone, of being cared for and connected. And you said when you went in as an adolescent, you did feel alone…?'

She reflects on the reasons for this, 'Yeah … I don't know if it's because I was more aware of what was going on. I think it was. They'd talk to *me* about the operation, so there was a different element that I hadn't been a part of before. And because I was more aware, it made me feel like I was more alone. I don't think I actually *was*, but I think there was that perception because *I* was the one actually dealing with it.'

In *Devotions upon Emergent Occasions*, John Donne[26] wrote, 'As Sicknesse is the greatest misery, so the greatest misery of sickness is solitude' (p. 30). I am curious about the nature of this aloneness, and want to tease out its meanings. It had echoes of Pat's experience and is certainly something that has resonance for me, as my questions increasingly reflect:

'So something about when you were actually living it, aware of it, and dealing with it brings home a sense of being ultimately alone?'

'Yes, it does. And even as a child going back to school, I felt a sense of responsibility; I've got to get on with it, I've got to do this. I remember feeling an aloneness. And I suppose those are the feelings that I have now.'

For Jan this is an embodied sense of being alone which is profoundly and inherently part of her life. So although she is not *by* herself, there was an almost existential aloneness when she 'is the one dealing with it'.

'YOUR HIPS AREN'T PERFECT'

By her late teens, Jan was having problems once again with her hips.

'I'd been discharged when I was 18. But when I was 19, my right hip started clicking again. So I went to see the surgeon … and he said, "Your hips aren't perfect", which dashed everything anyway. I didn't think they *were* perfect, but I didn't want to think they were imperfect in any way. But then he said, "You'll need them replaced in your late 30s." And I just thought, my god … I came away and I thought, I don't want to go back into a medical arena with it, because I don't want to meet people like that who don't have the time to say, "I know this might be quite difficult, but there are things we can do …" It was just "this is inevitable", and I don't think it should be. I didn't feel in a position to say to him, "Can you tell me something positive?" I didn't feel able to question him or anything. And that was topped by the fact that he presented it in an inevitable way … the possibility of trying different things was just taken away.'

Jan wanted recognition that she is a human being and that this was difficult for her. In conversation with Rita Charon, Jerome Bruner[27] tells the story of an eye operation and of one particular nurse who '*recognised* my human plight and shared it with me.' He goes on to say, 'My nurse recognised the fact that I was not just a "patient", I was somebody with plights, a human being' (p. 5).

Jan was also suggesting that it would have been preferable for her surgeon to have talked in terms of possibilities rather than finality and inevitability. Bruner[28] refers to anthropologist Byron Goode, who talks of the 'subjunctivisation of illness, something that physicians do for their patients that can give them considerable comfort by putting them in a twilight zone' (p. 8). The use of language in the subjunctive, employing phrases such as 'might be', or 'could be' then offers possibilities rather than conclusions; as Charon[29] says, 'by sidestepping the need for finality' we let 'everyone slowly absorb it, if it were to come to pass' (p. 9). If Jan's surgeon had tried to empathise with her, to sense her experience of hearing such finality and inevitability, perhaps Jan would have felt—to paraphrase Bruner above—recognised in her plight as a human being.

THE MOST DIFFICULT THING

The sense of inevitability Jan is presented with reminds her of the cycle of hospitalisation that dominated her childhood:

'That was when I started to think more about the surgery I'd had when I was younger and hoping that I didn't go through a repeating pattern—an ongoing process that would take over my life. Because I did feel it was no longer a huge part of my life, having got through the childhood stages of, "What are those scars?", and having to explain it, and it not being an issue. So at 19, to hear I would be going back into it … it was the surgeon who'd been involved in my last operation, and I felt that sense of him seeing me as a child. And that felt very awkward … I'd just finished my first year at university. I'd moved away. So it was really significant that I was going to see this man with my dad … this surgeon who was talking to me about my childhood difficulties when I'd just broken away. I think that was probably the most difficult thing, and it wasn't even about the surgery.'

Jan had started to live an independent life, and on the cusp of adulthood had been plunged into a situation which had powerful echoes of her dependent life as a child: echoes of disruption, and also of separation.[30] She was at a stage in her life when, in terms of Erikson's[31] psychosocial model of development, she was leaving the dependency of childhood and moving towards the establishment of a clear and independent sense of identity. Yet here she was, at 19, hearing that not only would she 'be going back into it', but that her hips were a defining characteristic of her identity.

THE HIP PROBLEM

'It felt like I was just the hip problem. I remember being younger and the doctors would never talk to me; they'd talk to my mum or my dad. There was that sense of *not* "I'm Jan", but "this is the hip problem". It felt like I was defined as that.'

Etymologically, the word 'define' derives from the Latin 'definire', meaning to limit, and its implication of determining a boundary. To experience a feeling of being 'defined' by a problematic body is diminishing for anyone. For Jan, at 19, it was particularly difficult; she was emerging from late adolescence, moving away from childhood dependency and into adulthood, where the establishing of independent identity is so important.

Frank[32] writes of how his diagnosis of cancer 'crowded out my name entirely. The hospital had created its own version of my identity. I became the disease, the passive object of investigation and later of treatment' (p. 52). Jan resists 'becoming the disease' or being defined by her condition.

'I think I've worked away from that, and now I don't think I *am* defined in that way. Whereas when I was younger, people were aware. If I fell over, it was, "Oh, Jan's hips", or "Should you be going skiing because of your hips?" It always entered into the equation somewhere. But it doesn't now—except in a way it does—but only to me. And I can hide that away.'

Jan has 'worked away from' being defined by her condition; it is something she 'can hide away', but at the same time its presence is inherently part of her life. From infancy she had a sense of her hips being problematic.

ALMOST BEING MAN-MADE

'I've had a sense of my bones being mended by other people; of them not being natural. I don't know how that makes me feel really. I've been thinking more and more about that sense of things not being right, and someone else having to make them better. Again the loss of control—helplessness really—over something that should be *so fundamental.*'

'I'm not sure here—but did you at times have the feeling of almost your body's not your own?' I wonder.

'I've always had that sense because of how it was described to me, that I was born with the ball and there wasn't a socket. So the doctors made you a socket, and they've had to keep on … So I've had a sense of almost being man-made. It's my body, but it has had to be shaped by somebody else. It's quite … and this is *fundamental* for me. It shouldn't have been. It should have been naturally OK. When my friends say, "Oh, you've got tiny hips", I'll be, "Yeah, but that's because they can't get any bigger." In terms of the impact upon my sense of me—*yes* in terms of the scars … Maybe the scars were an issue, though not so much now. But it probably would be if I was going on holiday. With people that I didn't know very well, I'd still be self-conscious of it—less so than I was. But then I grew up with that feeling that I needed to explain the scars to people; knowing that people are looking and wondering.'

Scars or disability are viewed as anomalies that require explanation. From childhood, Jan was 'different'; in adulthood, her scars mark that difference. As Couser puts it; 'In everyday life, for example, the unmarked case—the "normal" body—can pass without narration; the marked case—the limp, the scar, the wheelchair, the missing limb—calls for a story. Thus, people with anomalous bodies are often required to account for themselves'[33] (p. 19). It is a 'need to explain' that I recognised well, and which informed my next response:

'And thinking, how much do I explain here, and how much do I *want* to explain here?'

'Yeah—I certainly know when I go and get my legs waxed, the lady always says to me, "Are those recent scars?" And I've noticed things like, around the beauty therapy room, new treatments for scars; and I know that I went through a stage in my late teens just after the last operation, and I'd go into Boots and they had this scar stuff … and wanting to just get rid of them. But I don't think that's in terms of wanting to get rid of what I'd been through. For me it just felt a case of wanting to get rid of something that *only I* had—and especially then, it was quite an issue.'

Like Pat, Jan's scars represent 'what I'd been through'; in a sense, they honour and bear witness to her suffering, but at the same time mark her out as the 'only' one.

'And I suppose in the normal course of things *that* part of you would be invisible, but when it's the summer it's harder to keep it hidden, and I guess that's quite a difficult thing—'cos in a sense it's sharing quite a deep part of you?' I say tentatively.

'Yes, it *is*. And it's quite interesting that people never know, and that's nice, 'cos it's being in a more powerful position than your hips. But one of our friends is an osteopath, and he'll say, "Oh you're not walking properly". He's very helpful, but he'll say, "I think you should go and see an osteopath". And I think, No, I'm alright, thank you. And to think that some people *do* know, without my talking about it, feels a bit intrusive in a way; like they know my secret and they shouldn't.'

THE PRESENT AND FUTURE

Jan talks about the recurrence of her hip problems and what this means for her: 'I've started to get hip problems again, so there's that sense of not wanting to go back to that.'

I respond from my own 'felt sense'.[34] 'The feeling I got there—and this is probably coming from my experience—was, 'Will this ever go away?' As I move into the present with my own resonance, Jan picks up on this and reflects on her current concerns and fears for the future:

'And I don't think it will … and I don't know how upset that makes me feel. I don't want it to interfere now. It interfered before … certainly now with hip problems, I'll kind of deny it. You know—I'm *not* going to the doctors, 'cos I *know* what they're gonna say … I'll just carry on. It's the feeling of not wanting to get back into that.'

'There's a book by Arthur Frank[35] in which he writes of the fear of "going back into" that other world. And in my experience, there is a sense of it being a world cut off from ordinary life.' I say.

'Yeah, I think it is, isn't it? And I think that's probably why I don't think about my experiences because I can see it happening again … and I don't really want to think about it,' she says.

'And I'm aware that we're talking about it and wondering how you feel about that?' I check.

'It's nice to share it with somebody who isn't gonna say, "I think maybe you should go and see the doctor", because sometimes that is not what you want to hear. You just want to be able to say it, as opposed to somebody offering their opinions.'

She reflects further on the implications of it 'happening again':

'If I *did* go, I can just see this pathway of having the initial surgery, then surgery on the other hip … then having to redo the first hip. A continuation … and that's something that I *don't* want. I feel a sense of unfairness—that I shouldn't have to be going through this now … 'cos it's on a different pathway to how I see my life. And I don't want them to meet. I don't want it to get in the way of my career or my family life.'

BACK IN THE SYSTEM—THAT 'BIG BROTHER THING'

'The surgeon said by the time I'm mid-30s, "You'll have to have a hip replacement". Well I don't want to approach the medical profession. But maybe I should … before things get too difficult for the more minor procedures? But I think a time will come when I'm gonna have to make that decision. My feeling is that if I were to enter back into it for minor surgery, I would be back in the system—going back for check-ups. They'd be keeping an eye on me, and I don't quite want that Big Brother thing yet with that sense of being in somebody else's hands.'

Being 'back in the system' is complicated, ambiguous and full of contradiction: it can create deeply ambivalent feelings. Dependency brings with it a certain safety and security, but also anxiety and a sense of helplessness, of 'being in someone else's hands'. Sacks[36] writes of his own experience as a patient, 'one had to regress, for one might indeed be as helpless as a child' (p. 128). But such regression also means passivity and loss of control, and raises broader questions of how, as a patient, one might find a way of retaining a sense of agency. Jan is at a stage in her life when she wants to make her own decisions, and have a sense of control and of agency in her own life:

'In one way it's quite safe and secure; if something's got to be done, then somebody will be there to make the decisions for you,' she comments. 'But in another sense—maybe it's because of where I am in my life—I don't want to get into a position where somebody else is making the decisions for me. I've got my plans, and they actually *don't* include having hip problems or having somebody else dictate what should happen.'

She reflects on the difference between when she was a child and her present situation. 'I suppose when I was younger, the hip problems were always a family problem, whereas *now* they're actually *my* problem, and that's a very different experience to being taken with your mum …'

This difference is ambiguous for Jan. As a child, her parents were mediating on her behalf, whereas as an adult, the responsibility for actively dealing with it is Jan's. She reflects on this:

'I think in some ways, it's quite empowering, 'cos mum will say, "Oh, are you having your hip problems?" and I won't tell her. I'll keep it to myself. But it's quite scary, because there's a sense of responsibility that it's up to you to seek the help. And ultimately, *you* are making the decision to go down that path. But I don't feel comfortable making that choice at the moment.'

I respond with my own resonance, 'And it's a hard choice to take—to voluntarily step into that other world,' which Jan picks up and affirms.

'Yes, and I think that is the point. For me, it's a sense of the choice being there, and that wasn't there when I was younger. Now there's the choice to go down a route that I don't want to go down, or to ignore but live with the symptoms and the pain; there *is* a sense of that ultimately lying with me.'

For Jan there is a powerful shift from her childhood experience, where others are making decisions and are responsible for her well-being—to adulthood, where the dictates of her body limit her choices, but where she has a greater sense of agency.

'And it feels like I'm almost on a seesaw, because as the pain increases, I think maybe I should go and see someone, but then I think, no. I don't want to go down that route, because in a sense my hips will again define me whereas I've been trying to define myself as everything other than that.'

'You talked about the pain—how would you describe the pain, and how you live with it?'

'I think now it's more painful than it was. Now it's always there—I've always tried to ignore it, and if it gets very bad, then I'll take a tablet, but until then … I won't let it stop me doing anything though. But it has had its good parts actually. I remember at school it was quite funny, doing things like the Duke of Edinburgh award scheme with my friends—it would always be an excuse to stop: "Jan's hips are hurting"; and it's still brought up now if we're doing something and no one wants to carry on doing it! So there was a lighter side to it—and I suppose in that sense I did use it, 'cos it wasn't hurting …!'

We both laugh. 'That sounds really useful!' I say. 'For me, it brought up a resonance of how illness can get you out of other things that you might not want–illness as a form of escape …'

'Yeah—I think that's right—I don't know if other people would see that or understand that, but there were always times when having hip problems was put to very good use!'

'But in terms of the pain—for me it's the significance of the pain, and if the pain is getting worse, then … I'm getting closer to having to think about …'

IT'S ALL OF ME

For Jan there is no easy escape from 'having to think about it', since, as she says, 'It's so much part of me as a person that it is in my genes. And so in that sense it is more difficult to get away from. It's not something like having an appendix taken out. It's all of me.'

The genetic nature of her condition is particularly pertinent in terms of her relationship with her mother, and also in terms of having her own children.

'It's really interesting, Viv, because after the last time we met I felt really guilty, and I thought, what's that about … and I know it's about not wanting to misrepresent mum and dad … because it's a hereditary thing, my mum particularly feels guilty. She didn't have any hip difficulties herself, but hip difficulties are within the family, so I am really aware of what I say because of the hereditary aspect. I wouldn't want to say to them, "My hips are causing me real problems at the moment," because there'd be panic.

'It's comforting to think that I can tell them, but I think I'd rather tell my dad 'cos he'd be quite pragmatic whereas I feel like I'd know how my mum would be feeling. It's quite interesting—we had some teaching about paediatrics the other day, and guilt is one of the most common feelings that they work with in children. In terms of future difficulties—and because it is hereditary—there are my feelings about my children, and of course then there is the issue of increasing her sense of guilt because she'll feel that she's the one that has put this on her grandchild.

'In terms of the genetic nature of it, I suppose it is something I have to accept and I do accept. But I just have this feeling—I can imagine myself having my first child and being very happy and then suddenly thinking, I hope I haven't done anything. People say things are much different now. Treatments are very quick. And because they know you've had these problems, they'll keep an eye on it … That's fine, but it doesn't change the fact that it will happen. And that sense of responsibility; more than likely it will affect my children. I know that medicine's moved on and there are ways of treating it. But there's still that sense of putting somebody else through it. And even though I don't see my experience as being negative, it wouldn't be something that I'd want to impose on somebody else. And I wouldn't want that guilt feeling that my mum's got.'

IT DEFINITELY SHAPED WHAT I WANTED TO DO

Oliver Sacks[37] writes of 'the paradox of disease' and its 'creative potential' (p. xii). The paradox of illness stories is that they can encompass meaning-making and creative transformation as well as meaninglessness and chaos. While acknowledging the difficulties inherent in her condition, Jan felt that it had not been solely negative.

When I see her next, I ask her about the relationship between her experiences and her choice of career.

'It's very corny,' she says, 'but I've always known that I wanted to help people; there was a part of me that wanted to do medicine, but the other part of me … there was absolutely no way. I wanted to do things in a more practical way, on a deeper level. I often felt that the surgeons' work was kind of superficial; they did their bit and left. I did some work experience in an operating theatre. And as it happened, there was an orthopaedic surgeon in there. I just remember watching him … it was like a different kind of butchery in a sense; the person lying on the operating table wasn't really a person. I don't blame them for not seeing that, because that's how they're trained; but there was definitely a sense of that person *not* being somebody's son, somebody's dad. And I remember thinking, god, you're naked and all these people standing round you; there was that lack of seeing the person there. I just remember feeling very uncomfortable with it. And I knew that wasn't what I wanted.'

We talk of power and vulnerability, of the ritual of the ward round, and the fleet of junior doctors staring at you in your underwear when your 'case' is presented:

'It's that feeling of powerlessness, isn't it?' Jan says. 'That people can just do that to you! I remember thinking, I just wish the ground would open up; so I sat there really quietly—not wanting to look at all these people looking at you in your pants.'

'Yes,' I say, 'and that is so disempowering. It's a very unequal position to be in, isn't it?'

I continue, 'I can remember when I had angiograms; I was in these theatre knickers, and when they put the catheter into your femoral artery, you are lying there really exposed, with a mass of people around you.'

She nods. 'It's quite a depersonalising process, isn't it? And then people say, "Oh they've seen it all before." That's another one isn't it!'

We laugh wryly at the clichés and sense of ritual humiliation.

Jan reflects on the effects of it all: 'I see most of it as having had a lot of positive consequences … I think it definitely shaped what I wanted to do. It encouraged a sense of empathy even at a very young age … it made me more aware of my own feelings and shaped my personality to some degree. It helped me to know what I wanted to do in terms of wanting to be a help in more ways than just the physical side of things … and I think maybe that reflects my feelings about the power dynamics—I would never want to have that power differential with somebody who was vulnerable.'

In having access to her own vulnerability, Jan is able to recognise how important that is in her relationships at work and more able to undercut those power dynamics and to empathise with others. She consciously chose a career that she felt had less of a power differential, and to work in a way in which any power imbalance is held in awareness:

'It's striking, isn't it?' she continues. 'Being a doctor is such a powerful position to be in, and being a patient is such an undermining position. At work, people come in to see me, not really knowing what they're doing there, or what a psychologist is. We'll talk about the referral process, and they'll say, "Well I went to see so and so, and then the next thing I knew, I got a letter from you." It is that "passiveness in the process", isn't it? And what you're asking people to commit to is so much if they're not motivated. If you're not "active within the process", it's difficult to sign up for something, isn't it?'

'Yes,' I say. 'And I think being "active within the process"—that's such a good phrase—is really important. It's interesting how, as a psychologist, your experience of having been in the patient position makes you value that.'

'I think how scary it is to be within the system and to know at some higher level people are talking about you or sending letters to each other; as a patient there is that sense of watching it all going on above you and not even having access to watch it properly,' she reflects.

We talk of how difficult it is being 'passive in the process', within a healthcare system where, in Foucault's[38] terms, the domains of knowledge and domains of power are inseparable.

'Certainly,' Jan reflects, 'as we're talking about it now—it reminds me very much of the traditional ward round and having a group of doctors talking about you at the end of the bed. I remember seeing these bundles of medical notes and just thinking, what's in there? And in the folder at the end of your bed, what's in there?'

'Yes,' I nod, 'and wanting to see it … it's really strange; literally this week this issue has come up for me. I had the results of an MRI scan—and it was fine—but my notes are in this big folder. So when you said that about the notes I got such a vivid picture!'

'Yeah,' she replies, 'and I think it would be interesting to see; there's a sense that you'd like everything to be transparent, and sometimes I have to balance that with the fact that I might not want to know. There are days when I notice the pain; I try to put it to the back of my mind. I wouldn't even take tablets because I think "I'm not admitting it to myself". And for me at the moment, "getting on with it" is the most adaptive way to cope.' She pauses. 'I know further surgery is going to happen, and that will have to be got through and overcome. It's interesting, isn't it, that voice: "you should count yourself lucky", "just get on with it and get over it". That's something I wouldn't do at work. I would be conscious of it, deliberately not saying anything. It's difficult to feel that things don't feel fair—the "why me?" embedded in the "I feel sorry for myself." But then you do have to balance it up. I *do* think in the job that I do, I see a lot of people … and I think, well things aren't that bad. There's that empathy; I like it when people are able to say, "Why is this happening to me?" So often, people don't say it. I just think, "Well of course you're allowed to feel like that." But that goes against the more dominant discourse of: "Pull yourself together, get on with it,"' she observes.

I drive home, negotiating the twists and turns of the winding roads, and reflect on the way 'get on with it' storylines can impact on our selves and our lives, and the implications of this for Jan's professional identity. While 'getting on with it' and 'putting it on the back burner' are adaptive ways of coping with a long-term condition, she is mindful of the cultural codes of behaviour she has internalised, and this awareness of them as potential judgements informs the values she brings to her work.

Bennet discusses the polarity of the patient-doctor archetype and suggests a doctor's experience of 'the wound', if it is held in awareness, has the potential for creative transformation. He writes, 'Acknowledging the patient pole of the doctor-patient archetype enables the doctor to allow the actual patient to be other than the passive recipient of medical care'[39] (p. 220). This awareness and transformation of 'the wound' clearly informs Jan's relationships with her clients.

REFERENCES

1. Edelman G. *Bright Air, Brilliant Fire: on the matter of the mind.* London: Penguin; 1992.
2. Rosenfield I. *The Invention of Memory: a new view of the brain.* New York, NY: Basic Books; 1988.
3. Spence DP. *Narrative Truth and Historical Truth: meaning and interpretation in psychoanalysis.* New York, NY: Norton; 1982.
4. Ibid.
5. Gendlin E. *Focusing.* New York, NY: Everest House; 1978.
6. Polanyi M. *Personal Knowledge: towards a post-critical philosophy.* Chicago, IL: Chicago University Press; 1974.
7. Polanyi M. *The Tacit Dimension.* Gloucester, MA: Peter Smith; 1983.
8. Rosenfield, op cit.
9. Etherington K. *Trauma, Drug Misuse and Transforming Identities.* London: Jessica Kingsley; 2008.
10. Etherington K. *Becoming a Reflexive Researcher: using ourselves in research.* London: Jessica Kingsley; 2004.
11. Gee J. A linguistic approach to narrative. *J Narrative Life Hist.* 1991; **1**: 15–39.
12. Richardson L. *Poetic Representation of Interviews.* In: Gubrium J, Holstein JA, editors. *Handbook of Interview Research: context and method.* Thousand Oaks, CA: Sage; 2001.
13. Bateson G. *Mind and Nature: a necessary unity.* New York, NY: Dutton; 1979.
14. Bruner J. *Making Stories: law, literature, life.* New York, NY: Farrar, Straus and Giroux; 2002.
15. Ibid.
16. Bruner J. *Actual Minds, Possible Worlds.* Cambridge, MA: Harvard University Press; 1986.
17. White M, Epston D. *Narrative Means to Therapeutic Ends.* New York, NY: Norton; 1990.
18. Bowlby J. *Attachment and Loss: attachment (Vol. 1).* New York, NY: Basic Books; 1969.
19. Bowlby J. *Attachment and Loss: separation, anxiety and anger (Vol. 2).* New York, NY: Basic Books; 1973.
20. Bradley S. Suffer the little children: the influence of nurses and parents in the evolution of open visiting in children's wards 1940–1970. *Int Hist Nurs J.* 2001; **6**(2): 44–51.
21. Jolley J. Separation and psychological trauma: a paradox examined. *Paediatr Nurs.* 2007; **19**(3): 22–5.
22. Young J. Changing attitudes towards families of hospitalized children from 1935 to 1975: a case study. *J Adv Nurs.* 1992; **17**(12): 1422–9.

23. Alaoui-Ismaïli, *et al.* Odor hedonics: connection with emotional response estimated by autonomic parameters. *Chem Senses.* 1997; **22**(3): 237.
24. Becker G. *Disrupted Lives: how people create meaning in a chaotic world.* Berkeley and Los Angeles, CA: University of California Press; 1999.
25. Ibid.
26. Donne J. *Devotions upon Emergent Occasions.* Ann Arbor, MI: University of Michigan Press; 1959.
27. Bruner J. *Narratives of Plight: A conversation with Jerome Bruner.* In: Charon R, Montello M. *Stories Matter: the role of narrative in medical ethics.* New York, NY: Routledge; 2002.
28. Ibid.
29. Ibid.
30. Spence, op cit.
31. Erikson E. *Childhood and Society.* New York, NY: Norton; 1950.
32. Frank A. *At the Will of the Body.* Boston, MA: Houghton Mifflin; 1991.
33. Couser T. *Disability as Metaphor.* In: *Prose Studies,* (1 and 2), pp. 141–52. Available at: www.informaworld.com/smpp/title~content=t713662173~db=all~tab=issueslist~branches=27 - v2727 (accessed 2005).
34. Gendlin op cit.
35. Frank A. *The Wounded Storyteller: body, illness and ethics.* Chicago, IL: University of Chicago Press; 1995.
36. Sacks O. *A Leg to Stand On.* Rev ed. London: Picador; 1991.
37. Sacks O. *An Anthropologist on Mars.* London: Picador; 1995.
38. Foucault M. *Power/Knowledge: selected interviews and other writings.* Gordon C, editor. New York, NY: Pantheon Books; 1980.
39. Bennet G. *The Wound and the Doctor: healing, technology and power in modern medicine.* London: Secker and Warburg; 1987.

CHAPTER 4

Jim's story

INTRODUCTION

Jim was in his early 40s when he had a heart attack. Angiography showed that his coronary arteries were blocked, and that he was in urgent need of a coronary artery bypass graft. The surgery was successful. On discharge from hospital, and after six weeks of rest and recuperation at home, he took part in a programme of cardiac rehabilitation and counselling. After a period of gradual re-integration into his job as a manager in a large supermarket, he was able to return to work full-time.

I DIDN'T SEE IT COMING

Jim's first telling of his story had a very clear shape. He introduced it with the words: 'my story's gonna be strange', which explicitly signalled the occurrence of the unexpected on which the narrative turns, and the beginning of a sequence of events in the past that extend into the present and open out to an anticipated future.

'It was like really strange, because I was fit and well … or I'd assumed I was. I *felt* fit and well; I used to walk, to ride a bike … maybe ate too much, maybe drank too much. And I just didn't see it coming. But most probably my wife did … or she had some inkling I wasn't 100 per cent.'

He explains here the reason why his story is 'strange', and hints at a sense of causality that implicitly indicates the plot of his story: a plot that hinges on an expectation of being 'fit and well'. His sense of surprise and shock reflects a world-view that associates heart disease with advancing age and decline in fitness (p. 71).[1]

A CERTAIN DAY

Jim then goes on to set the scene by locating his story within a particular location, a personal and social context and along a temporal dimension.[2]

'I went to work on a certain day … and I was actually suspended from work for a misdemeanour. I was asked to go home and take a couple of days leave with pay … it was something and nothing … basically an ex-manager called in … I took him into the restaurant, got him a cake, bought him a cup of tea. I thought that was the professional thing to do. And the manager at the time didn't think that was right; she told me to go home and she'd call me in a couple of days' time—which I thought really was ok.'

The beginning of his story rapidly raises expectations of a shift from the normality of 'going to work'; as soon as we read or hear the words 'certain day', we know this is not *any* working day; we anticipate the occurrence of the unexpected. Jim continues by describing the circumstances in which he experienced the onset of his symptoms. Implicit in the start of Jim's story, then, is the sense that this is not just an ordinary day at work. There is a sense that his suspension from work, though not in itself a serious occurrence, has a bearing on what is to follow.

A PRESSING PAIN

The occurrence of the unexpected—the symptoms that follow (both in a temporal sense, and— perhaps to a degree—in a causal sense) quickly turn the series of events into a story. Jim's sense of order in the world, which has been disturbed by events at work, is further disrupted when he starts to experience chest pain.

'But when I come home, I had like a pressing pain here—like something continuously pressing on my chest. My arm was a bit achy at the top and I didn't feel right. So Louise, my wife, works in a clinic which is walking distance—so I walked down and one of the nurses said, "You all right?" And I said, "Yeah, but I got this pain in me shoulder and me arms." And she said, "Let me do your blood pressure", and said it was a bit high, nothing to worry about, and that I should see the doctor. So that's what I did. And the doctor said, "Just take it easy for a couple of days. Any further problems, just give me a ring."'

Jim's story involves his wife's observations and interventions from the very beginning: his feeling that she may have 'had some inkling', and the implicit sense that he saw a doctor because his wife worked at the clinic nearby. This reflects the often-reported gender differences in use of health services, such as men delaying seeking help.[3,4]

TESTS

The symptoms represent a significant bodily change that precipitates a sequence of events transforming the ordinary and everyday of Jim's life into the extraordinary and unexpected: the world of medical tests.

'And just as I was leaving—I was actually outside the surgery—she popped her head round and said, "Will you just have an ECG for me?" And she was like persistent, so I went back in. And it was getting worse. The technician give me the ECG, and then went out and seen the doctor. "Oh," she said, "There's something wrong with the machine. I'll just go and get the doctor to check it."

'And when they come back in, she said, "Oh, you've had a heart attack." And I said, "When?!" And she said, "Not long ago." And off I went—they bundled me straight into hospital. I spent a couple of days and I had different tests done. And they said I needed to take a treadmill test, and I said, "Fine, no problem." So we went home and waited.'

The continuum between Jim's personal experience and its sociocultural context is exemplified by the urgency of events and initial tests; the incident at work, the occurrence of symptoms, the ECG and news that it was a heart attack (the personal) are followed by a long delay in which Jim 'went home and waited' (the sociocultural).[5]

'This went on for about a month, and then my wife rang up and said, "My husband's fixed up this treadmill test and we're a bit concerned—it's been about four weeks." And they said, "Well we've got no record of him ever coming into this hospital." And my wife said, "No, he was in there for two days and he had a heart attack." At the time I was still playing golf, and I'm just like carrying on with life normally. And Louise badgered them—she phoned up virtually every day—and they said, "We've found it; it was on a Post-it on the back of his notes. Can you come out today?" So we went out.'

The speed and immediacy of the initial diagnosis is in sharp contrast to waiting for a month. Jim carries on as normal, putting to one side the disruption of the heart attack. With the support and intervention of his wife, the note referring Jim for a treadmill test is eventually located, and he undergoes the test.

'I gotten on the treadmill … I was on the treadmill for about 15 seconds, and I was all wired up, and she said, "Stop. You need to stop, you've got a problem." And I said, "What? It feels fine." She said, "You have to stop now. You have to take these beta-blockers. Just go home, sit in the chair, and do nothing. We'll tell you when you need to have an angiogram." And that's what I did.'

The circumstances of such delays where diagnosis and treatment hinge on a note that 'goes missing' give us information about the social and political context of the National Health Service (NHS) in the United Kingdom in 2002. After a month of waiting, of not knowing, of finding a way of 'carrying on with life normally' while 'a bit concerned', the outcome of the treadmill test shows Jim 'how serious it was' and he decides to 'go private'.

'Once we realised there was summat up, we went from NHS to private. At first I'd thought it was going to be taking tablets. But once I realised how serious it was, I thought now is the time to go private. And I was lucky enough to have quite good medical insurance from the company I work for. So with the insurance I've got through my company—who were fantastic—I was put in touch with a doctor and I went up for the angiogram. I was still thinking, "Naa, everything will be alright."'

THINKING I WAS BULLETPROOF

The dramatic tension of Jim's story powerfully reflects the 'peripeteia' which 'swiftly turns a routine sequence of events into a story'[6] (p. 5). The deviation from the ordinary, everyday routine of life to the extraordinary, and unexpected, is highlighted in his vivid description of the angiogram and ensuing diagnosis: in this he draws on a wide range of evocative metaphors from contemporary United Kingdom culture, which I discuss further in Chapter Six.

'I went up and had the angiogram on the Monday in the January. That was weird—it was done in the back of a lorry. I was lifted up; it was like going into the Tardis—televisions were everywhere.[7] And the thing that stuck in my head was—do you know that feeling when you get a plumber come and he'll like tap your radiator and go, "tut tut ... ooh." Sharp intake of breath ... eyes up in the air. And this doctor, I shall never forget—I'm useless with names but I'll always remember him. He had all the gear on and all of a sudden, all of these screens just come alight, and he looked and he went, "Oh, that's no good." He said, "You need a bypass; that artery is blocked ... that one's blocked ... you got many of them blocked there." And I went back in the room, and I was really upset—obviously thinking I was bulletproof, and gonna live forever. The guy who was gonna do the operation come and see me a couple of hours later and he said, "You need a bypass. I can do it, and we'll do it in March or April."'

This powerful description shows the rapid shift from the order and routine of 'carrying on normally' to the shock and major disruption of a diagnosis of a serious heart condition that requires surgery.

TREATMENT

Later that day, when Jim reached home, there was a call from the hospital to say they would prefer to operate as soon as possible and that this could be done in a few days' time. With the agency and encouragement of his wife and his sister, Jim agreed to the surgery. He swiftly recounts the urgency of events:

'My sister come over to see how I was, and the phone went and it was the hospital. They said, "We'd rather see you sooner than later. The surgeon has a gap on Thursday of this week," and I was like, "No." And my sister said, "Say yeah. Say you'll do it". And I said, "I'll ring you back." So I rang my wife, and she come straight out. "Right what are we going to do?" she said. And I said, "Well we've got to have it done Thursday". She said, "Well do it then—no time to worry about it." And that's what we done. So it was like angiogram Monday, operation on the Thursday. I was back out the following Friday.'

As he told the story with its clear beginning, middle and end, there was no need—nor would it have been appropriate—to ask questions. In subsequent conversations with Jim, there were opportunities to follow up some of the stories touched on in this first over-arching narrative.

The coherence of Jim's first telling of his story reflects the clear trajectory of the 'restitution narrative'[8] with its progression from symptoms to tests and diagnosis to treatment and recovery; while his account reflects the shape and plot of the 'restitution' narrative, it also contains elements of 'chaos' and of the beginning of meaning-making implicit in the quest narrative. The pace of his story reflects something of the pace of events that followed the angiogram; the speed with which this all happened meant that Jim barely had time to take it in.

NO TURNING BACK

When I next saw Jim, I asked him about his experience in hospital.

'My daughter and my wife took me up on the Thursday morning, early doors; I was in there for half seven. They give me a razor and said I had to shave my body; it was a funny sort of razor, like a woman's razor, but it was really good. And then the anaesthetist come in, and we had a little chat and he told me exactly what happens. Then the surgeon come in and told me exactly what he was going to do, bit by bit. And then they give me like a calming pill, I suppose it was—a chill-out pill—and I just took that and I went drowsy and woozy. I asked if I could walk, and they said, "No, you can't walk," and they sat me down on the bed … and then they wheeled me down.'

'Can you remember what your feelings were around that time …?' I ask.

'Fear … fear. But once I got into the lift and the lift went down, the fear seemed to go … because there was no turning back, you know? I couldn't go back. You know?'

I nod. I do know. As he describes the fear that is sublimated by a form of steely resignation, I am taken back in my head to my own experience. I remember a kind of respite that comes with that sense of 'no going back', and also a sense of 'the only way through this is through this'. And I attend closely as he retraces his own journey from the pre-op procedures to the 'no turning back' stage.

He continues: 'And then I can remember, when I was in the lift, like really fighting to keep my eyes open, trying to stay awake, although I hadn't been anaesthetised, as yet. I was aware of what was going on around me, but I weren't really awake. I knew people were speaking to me, and the anaesthetist come in and said, "I'm going to put something into your arm now, and you'll feel a tingling and I want you to count backwards from 10, like 10, 9, 8 …" I can remember doing that. Then I remember waking up and being really freezing cold, and I can remember someone speaking to me … they must put you in some sort of waiting corridor … and dropped the temperature down, maybe to stop you bleeding … but it was freezing … and I can remember being in this like cold metal trailer, like a body shape. That's what it felt like. I didn't know where I were.'

'That must have been quite a weird feeling, quite disorientating …' I say.

'Yes. 'Cos I could see like the masks and the people around, and they was talking to me. I was answering as well. They were saying, "Are you alright, Jim? Just relax." And then nothing. The lights went out.'

As Jim describes the detail of losing consciousness, I think of how this story is so often *not* told; so many people, wheeled down to the operating theatre, so many different feelings. I think of how we have to surrender control and to place trust in those who will be caring for our unconscious bodies.

COMING ROUND

'And then I can remember … it seemed like warmth, I suppose. I was coming round and there was this old nurse, and she was lovely. She went, "Hello, I've been waiting for you." And she said, "Would you like a drink?" … and I was so dry. And she got me about that much water and a straw and I thought I'd been restrained somehow … I couldn't get up. I could lift my head, but I couldn't get up. She give me this drop of water.'

Pat had talked of nursing as an art, and I can see how Jim's nurse with her warmth and humanity lived that art with her patients; like Bruner's nurse, who 'recognised my human plight'[9] (p. 5).

'And I can remember I started to cough, and I'd think, "best not cough." I was 24 hours in intensive care. I can't remember seeing my wife … I can remember waking up at different times and them putting something in my mouth like a wet sponge. It tasted horrible … like polystyrene. I didn't like it at all, but she kept doing it, and then I just kept falling in and out of consciousness. I didn't feel as though I was sleeping. I felt as though they was giving me something to keep me sedated.

'On the Saturday, they said we're going to take me to HDU (High Dependency Unit). I had a nurse during the day for 12 hours, and she was a big old girl; she was lovely, really lovely. I remember when they lifted me up, I started feeling sick, and she said, "Try to eat something". She went away, and she come back and she give me little small squares of dry bread, and the sickness went away straight away and within 10 minutes … quarter of an hour, I was quite happy for the family to come in. I knew I wasn't like 100 per cent 'cos I had tubes and tubes. That must have been on Sunday evening …'

As Jim tries to piece together this period from just before anaesthesia to recovering consciousness and being moved to HDU, he is relocating himself along a temporal axis, and in Ricoeur's sense, 'time becomes human'[10] once again; I remember piecing together that same period of my own experience, and a sense it was important to do so, because otherwise it was a gap; a period of 'no-time'. Pat had talked to me of the 'emptiness of anaesthesia' and of it being 'like a little death'; this was both from her perspective as a patient, and as a nurse in theatre, when she experienced the person under general anaesthetic as 'becoming a body, not a person'. In relocating ourselves before and after anaesthesia, we are in a sense reclaiming a sense of personhood from that 'gap'.

He continues. 'Then when I moved from HDU, I was quite frightened, because there you got one-to-one care …'

'There's always someone there, isn't there?' I say.

'Yes, someone there … someone to talk to … And then I was taken out of HDU and put in the next room. Then, to my surprise—because I didn't realise—they said, "Now we're gonna remove the catheter today." I thought, "I've got a catheter!" I didn't know! But they removed it and boy, is that painful! Just for that instant. And I think I was still sedated a bit, because it was a bit surreal. And then I went through a stage of about 24 hours when I couldn't stop crying, and I couldn't understand … my mum come and seen me on the Monday or Tuesday and I just could not stop crying. I couldn't say it was because I was watching the telly—I think I was watching EastEnders … and it was so sad, I cried my eyes out. I spent like about 12 hours, and my sister, my brother-in-law and my mum come in. My wife had to keep taking me to the bathroom, because I was still a bit unsteady on my feet; not that I wanted the toilet—but just so I could compose myself a little bit. I couldn't understand why I was crying. And then afterwards, the cardiac nurse come in, and she said, "Yes, you will feel like that, that's all part and parcel of it. It's like someone's made a massive assault on your body." And I felt like that for about 12 hours. But that was all.'

A BIG BARRIER

'And after that it all seemed to move very quickly. Some young Australian physio-therapist come in, pulled the curtain and said, "Out you get then!" and I was like …! And she said, "Come on." And I went, "Come on what then?" She said, "Get out," and I said, "No … no. I just had a by-pass!"

Oliver Sacks[11] reflects on the symbolism of standing and walking, and writes: 'Rising, standing, walking pose for every bed-ridden patient a fundamental challenge, for he has forgotten, or been disallowed the adult, human posture and motions of uprightness, that physical-and-moral posture', and notes that it is, 'moral, existen-tial, no less than it is physical' (p. 98).

'They get you moving straight away, don't they?' I say, remembering the impor-tance of the physiotherapists' encouragement to resume an upright adult posture.

'Yeah, and I couldn't move. I mean, I couldn't get out of bed to go to the toilet. And she said "Up!" And I'm like, "Whoah … I'm not going anywhere." I said, "How am I going to get up with bits and pieces hanging out of everywhere?" She went, "Use the rope on the end of the bed," and I'm looking at her and I'm like, "No way!" He laughs. 'But, um, no, she just kept on … She said, "Get out of bed, you can go to the bathroom by yourself, you can wash by yourself, you can come home." So I pulled myself up on this rope and swing my legs round. And course, you don't know …'

'You're wobbly, aren't you?' I say.

He nods. 'You're really wobbly on your feet. Once I was sat on the bed, I was like giddy and … But she said, "Come on", and I said, "Where are we going?" And she said, "Well, I thought we'd go down the corridor". And she walked me 10, 15 paces there and 15 paces back. That was a big barrier, because you think to yourself, "Right, I did that by myself."'

I respond with my own resonance, 'It sounds like—and I remember this too— you almost don't have the confidence to do it. You almost have to have somebody saying, "Right, you can do this now," don't you?'

'Yes, that's it. And I was really frightened … walking was scary. Then the next day you walk, say 30 steps, and then back, and then the next day you walk a bit further.

She would come back in every so often and say, "Come on, shall we go for a walk?" And then, after a bit you're waiting for her to come back in, so we actually bonded, you know? First off, I didn't really care for her, but it was like we really bonded. She used to come in and switch the golf on, and we watched the golf and then she'd say, "Come on, shall we see if we can go to the cafeteria?" And we'd shuffle along very, very slowly.'

Again, Jim experiences both the *art* and the *heart* of nursing; a quality of care which contributes so much to the process of recovery, of regaining strength and building confidence in fragile bodies. His nurse and physiotherapist are maintaining a delicate balance of physical and psychological holding and supporting, as well as pushing and encouraging him towards independent walking and 'being'.

A MASSIVE FIRST

'Another thing that really frightened me was—when I first went on the ward—I could hear people coughing, and I thought, God, if you cough, your chest must like explode … especially at this stage, 'cos I'd still got this piece of gauze down here and it's taped. So it was tight, but I didn't know if I had stitches or what was underneath that.

'It was like everything was a massive first. Just before I come out, the big old nurse who used to look after me—she was smashing, she was—she said, "I bet you'd like a shower and a shave." And I said, "Would I ever?" She said, "Why not?" I said, "Well, I got this dressing on …!" And she shuffled me over, sat me in the shower and she shaved me. Then she washed me and she just pulled it off. And I was like, "No!" And when she pulled it off, there was no stitches. In fact, it was just like a red scar. No stitches at all!

'I was like … I mean, I couldn't touch it. I couldn't wash it. She had to wash it, and it was like so clean it was untrue, like no nasty stuff. I was expecting loads of stitches. And all I had was three stitches across the bottom. It was really weird. And when I come home and had showers I couldn't bear to wash … I couldn't touch it. I couldn't look at it. Although like now, no problem at all, but at the time, I couldn't even look at it,' he repeats.

The thought of seeing his wound mirrors and represents the 'massive first' of encountering the fallibility of his body. Its exposure is too much to contemplate; it signifies the frailty and fragility of his body and the confrontation with his mortality.

'The next stage was a woman coming in to reinflate the lung, 'cos my lung had been collapsed as well; you got to suck into this tube thing and it raises three balls. You got to try to get all three of them up. And that was really painful, but the physiotherapist got me through that as well. She was only young, but she seemed to know her stuff; she seemed to be switched on and knew what she was doing.'

'It's interesting; they know what you can do, and how far to push you. That sort of helps build your confidence up, doesn't it?' I say.

'Yes, they sort of push you and push you.'

THEN COME THE TERRIBLE DAY

With the support and encouragement of nurses and physiotherapists, Jim is in a position to offer support to one of his fellow patients:

'When I was on the ward, this nurse come in, and she said, "There's a guy next door, and he is really frightened. Can you go and have a chat to him?" And I said, "Right, yeah, sure." So I went and had a chat with this guy, and he was like really pleased. And we bonded a little, 'cos we spent a couple of days together.

'And then come the terrible day when they say, "Right, you can go home." The surgeon come in and said, "You can go home. It's time to go home." And I didn't want to go ... I said, "I don't want to go home. In here, if I get a pain, you give me a tablet and I'm fine ..." Do you know what I mean?' he asks me.

I say, 'I understand that. There's someone you can ask. You feel very vulnerable, don't you, when you go out?'

'Yes, and all the technology's around ... although I *was* looking forward to going home.'

'Yes, absolutely,' I say, affirming my shared understanding of the apparent contradiction involved in relinquishing support and care, while also looking forward to returning home.

'And the fear factor's gone by then. I'd come through six or seven days, and I could see how I was getting stronger and my brain was thinking quicker. I had bad dreams, though. Really weird dreams.'

Even though 'the fear factor' has gone, it surfaces in Jim's dreams. I ask him about these.

'I couldn't really explain them. Not really frightening dreams. Just really strange. I can remember one night the nurse coming in, and I was stood by the window. And the next morning she said, "I was having a conversation with you last night in your sleep. And you was on about the trees out there and you were going to go out and climb the trees." Obviously I couldn't get out, 'cos all the windows were shut,' he adds. 'They were weird dreams—like hallucinating, I should imagine. You know, like big spiders. And coming home was really frightening ... and also, it was very emotional leaving all the people ...'

'The other patients?' I ask.

'Yes, and also your nurses, 'cos your nurses are 24-7, so you have the same nurse almost every day. You share books and cards and boxes of chocolates with people, and it was very emotional; it was like cuddles, and really emotional. And I didn't want to go 'ome. But I *did* want to go 'ome. But it was hard, and a bit scary. And also you've formed these strong bonds with people as well, haven't you?' he says, referring to my understanding of the complexity and ambiguity of this particular form of 'separation anxiety'.[12]

'I remember coming out and feeling quite anxious about leaving the security of the hospital. But at the same time, desperate to come home ...' I say.

'Yet not wanting to leave,' he adds, completing the sentence. 'I can remember after the first few days on the ward; I had a lump—I think it was because I was sitting -and one of the nurses used to massage me. She'd put the telly on and say, "Do you want a cup of tea or some chocolate?" and she'd go off and make me some ...' He smiles as he remembers these acts of care and kindness. 'Then they said, "Just go home, sit in the chair and do nothing. Six weeks. Just come home, don't do anything." And that's what I done!'

At this point, Jim neatly ties up the end of this first part of his story. His sense of order has been ripped apart by the speed and immediacy of events; the confrontation with death that his heart disease has represented, the massive disruption to his sense of order and of his previously embodied self leave him with nothing to do but to 'go home' and 'sit in the chair'. This period of immobilisation is an enormously difficult one. The instructions are to be passive, and to 'do nothing'. But, as Becker[13] (p. 46) writes:

> People who experience the sudden onset of a chronic illness face the destruction of life itself, the destruction of the habituated embodied self, as well as uncertainty about whether they have time to create themselves anew. They are immersed simultaneously in addressing the possible end of their lives and learning how they will manage in daily life if they live.

The 'massive firsts' Jim experienced in hospital: his first tentative steps, the initial shock of encountering his wound, his discharge and return home, all reflect the breaking apart of his previous sense of a whole healthy body and the life expectations which accompany that.

I ask Jim about this period of 'sitting in the chair for six weeks'.

'Well, it was OK. I was quite happy to do that. I felt like safe being in the house.'

In emerging from the hospital world into the safety of home, he starts the process of adjusting to the disruption to his everyday life and expectations of what and how his life would be. This period of initial convalescence and of gradual reentry into the outside world is one in which Jim is supported by family and friends.

'Home was safe; I mean, they wouldn't let me go too far. I was only allowed to walk round the green ... 'cos we did have one incident where we went down the village and we parked, and I went to get the ticket. It was important to me that I got the ticket, and when I got to the machine it wasn't working, and the next machine was up an incline. So off I set, and about half way I run out of steam. Literally I just buckled, and that frightened me and Louise, my wife. It was like Christ, what's going on? And then we sat on the wall, and she went and got the car and we had to come home. And I stayed there. I just sat. And Louise and the kids got me Sky Sports. But you know, there's only so much sport you can watch in one day. I read books and played a bit and just didn't do anything for six weeks …'

The first time I had met Jim, I had noticed and commented on his guitar, which stood in the corner of the room. I told him I used to play, and immediately he talked about how much he enjoyed music; when I asked him what songs were particularly significant for him, he picked up the guitar and played 'Redemption Song'.[14] Bob Marley had written that song around the time he was diagnosed with the cancer from which he died in 1981; the poignancy and beauty of his solo acoustic recording told a story of slavery and suffering, of struggle for freedom. It was a song of freedom and redemption, which, now 25 years later, held meaning and resonance for Jim as he emerged from the world of illness. As I had listened to Jim play, I'd heard the sound of a man appreciating freedom and deliverance from the world of sickness; the freedom to rebuild a life; a freedom he could not have been sure of finding again. I heard his recognition of how precious that sense of 'redemption' is alongside the uncertainty and doubt that illness leaves in its wake.

I thought of the contradictions inherent in surviving life-threatening illness and remembered how, about a week after my surgery, I had experienced a flash of realisation that I was alive with the possibility of a future and the chance to see my children grow up. It came to me like a blinding revelation; it was joyous and exhilarating. With that initial euphoria came a sense of release and liberation. But, like Jim, I experienced intense vulnerability and anxiety alongside that freedom, and felt an enormous and indescribable fear that 'it' could happen again. A sense of uncertainty had taken residence, which had descended on my body from the moment of diagnosis, and it was no longer possible to take my health for granted. Like Jim, I needed the solace and comfort of home and close family; a chance for my body and spirit to begin to heal. I needed time to take in the reality of what had happened and to mourn the loss of my life before illness.

I reflected on how challenging and ambiguous it had been for him to recover from an illness that went literally and metaphorically to the heart of his being. He had talked about the emotion and the fear he had experienced on leaving hospital; he was delighted to be going home, but also anxious about leaving the security of the hospital and all it represented in terms of care, knowledge and expertise.

THAT WAS THE FEELING OF FEAR

'I can remember just coming home and that was really like *it*. *That* was the feeling of fear; when you're in hospital, you've got everything there, so if you have a twinge there's a doctor or a nurse there straight away. That first week or fortnight …' he pauses. 'Good grief … I'd think, What is gonna happen to me? What's gonna happen from here on? And there were certain barriers and certain things … like I went through all the emotions ... of like closing my eyes and being frightened to go to sleep because I might not wake up again. Do you know what I mean?' he asks me.

'Yes ...' I nod. 'My memory of that period was of feeling, "What is my life gonna be? What does this mean for my life?" And at that point, when you've just come out of hospital, you actually don't know, do you?'

'No, you don't. Once you've been to the edge ... the most horrifying thing for me was not necessarily the operation; I was quite OK with that. I think I handled that and the aftermath pretty well. I was like the model patient. I got the booklet and it would say, "Right, on Day One you'll walk to the gate"; so Day One I walked to the gate. "On Day Two you go up to the telegraph pole" ... but there were times just after my heart attack when I thought, I'm not gonna make old bones. Do you know what I mean?'

'Oh I do.'

'We used to talk at length—me and Louise, 'cos she stayed home for two weeks and looked after me. I was really apprehensive when she went back to work. I didn't like that first day. But I had so many people calling in ... just an endless stream, which was really cool, bringing me magazines and DVDs and giving me a chance to think about things. So I didn't used to spend a lot of time on my own.

'And it was really touching all the people in work who cared for me. I didn't realise how people cared; they used to come out quite regularly. There were two managers used to ring up regularly, and I remember one come out with a bouquet of flowers, and I thought, that's a funny thing to bring out for a bloke, and I said, "They're not for me?" and he goes, "They're for your wife, 'cos we knows what she's gotta put up with, 'cos you're a miserable so-and-so!" But really thoughtful; not only thinking about what I was going through but obviously what the family was going through. And you need that to get through troubled times; you need the support of your family, and I had total support—not necessarily wrapped up in cotton wool, but I could see they were all concerned and worried.'

Sacks[15] writes of being discharged after his leg injury: 'The sheer complexity and bustle of the world was terrible' (p. 129). Jan had talked of her return to school as 'feeling like I'd had my cotton wool ripped off from around me'. I had written of my own experience of emerging from the dependency and confinement of illness into the outside world; 'the prospect of emerging from a state of utter dependence and powerlessness was daunting ... I was as vulnerable as I had ever been in my life'[16] (p. 143). Daunting as it is to emerge from the 'cotton wool' of the institution that is hospital, it is equally daunting to take the next step out of the world of convalescence into the social world. And it was this stage of Jim's recovery that I was curious about.

'The first six months were tough. It was like everything was a massive first; like going to the golf club for the first time. Louise dropped me off, and I felt fine. And then—whether I had a panic attack or what, I don't know—but I got a terrible stomach ache. I was on the putting green, but I couldn't concentrate, I was in so much pain. And I told my friend, and he said, "Don't worry; I'll take you straight home."

I thought I was having a panic attack. 'Nurse' Louise used to make me go to sleep every afternoon … we got into a bit of a pattern … we found it worked better if I went up about one o'clock and just had like an hour's kip. Then I could keep going till about nine or 10 o'clock at night.'

REHABILITATION

'The big kick was when we went to cardiac rehab, and we both had to go, and the nurses there were absolutely superb. The next week I went back on my own, and I met up with two other guys. We'd all had heart bypasses … and we did strike up a relationship straightaway. While we did our exercises, we'd sit and talk; someone would say, "Do you get a pain?" "Yes. Do you?" … and so on. And as we all done our rehab, we was monitored up. There were nurses there and always one who'd be like the governor; she was walking round and if she seen somebody who was short of breath, she'd stop and check. So we had about five or six sessions together, which was good.

'And then one day they took us for a walk along the sea wall and the Downs. That was nice. We all marched all the way over there; then marched all the way back. In the afternoon, we used to have sandwiches and fruit. Then we'd have relaxation, which was pretty good. And nine times out of 10 someone would fall asleep; one of us would hear snoring in the background! And then every day they'd bring some-one in: one time we had a doctor; then we had a nutritionist and they took us to a supermarket and told us what food to look out for.'

COUNSELLING

'And then Carole, the counsellor, come in one day and spoke to us. First off, I thought I didn't need counselling. When she first came in, I was thinking, "boring", and then she said, "This is how you'll feel now, and most probably in a couple of weeks' time you'll feel depressed and teary", and I thought, "No, not me". But like whatever she said it seemed to be 'appening. Like, after a couple of weeks, I could have cried me eyes out, and I'm not a crying person. Then she said I'd go through the angry stage. And that come later—like "Why me?" She'd tell us what to expect. And she was dead right. Like I used to find it difficult to say "no" to things; like if I was in work and there was a job that needed to be done that weren't very nice, I'd say, "I'll do it". Or if one of the kids said, "Oh can you pick me up from town at say two in the morning?" I'd say, "Yeah", and I'd be on at work say six till two tomorrow; and I'd say, "Oh it's all right, I'll manage." And so one of the big things getting me head round was saying no.'

Jim found these sessions enormously beneficial: they seemed to bring a sense of order and shape to the disorder, chaos and shock of heart disease. It was a context in which experience could be shared, thus creating connection in place of the isolation that serious illness can bring. His relationship with the other men allowed discussion of shared concerns, in an atmosphere of trust where they had access to information and advice. In addition, he became aware of his own patterns of behaviour, and of setting his own boundaries. Thus, rehabilitation offered a bridge—a kind of halfway house and a means of transition between the world of illness and everyday life.

The concept of rehabilitation—the restoration and facilitation of people to optimal physical and mental health—developed out of the recognition in the early 20th century of the effects of physical impairment[17] (pp. 27–47). The original emphasis of rehabilitation was on the physical impact of illness and disability, and rehabilitation principally involved exercise as a means of preparing people for return to work. The concept evolved and grew to include psychological intervention and support in both physical and mental health.[18]

In a review of cardiac rehabilitation, Hession[19] found the primary focus was on 'rebuilding physical strength' with 'little evidence of appropriate psychological intervention despite the incidence of depression and its link with cardiac mortality' (p. 17). However, Jim was fortunate to experience rehabilitation that offered both psychological as well as physical support.

WALKING THROUGH THE DOOR

'The first six months were tough, though. The company I work for were absolutely fantastic at the time; they put together a fantastic programme, and they didn't put any pressure on me to come back to work. They said, "We'd like you to come back next week, but just come in for half an hour." So I started going back for half an hour a week, then it went to four hours a week, then eight hours, and I could choose what days I wanted to go in.'

'So how did that feel—going through that process? And what did it feel like when you first went back to work?'

'When I first went back, it was horrendous. I was terrified just walking through the door. Just opening the door and going in. Once I got through, I was OK, but the first time was awful. It's like everything seemed to be a first. Driving to work—massive; walking back through the doors—massive; being introduced to new people—massive ... 'cos obviously after six months people come and people go. So I had new managers; it was all like new people.'

'The door' represented a kind of threshold[20] between the world of illness and the world of work, and 'walking through' it signified the magnitude of the transition, or 'rite de passage', between those worlds.[21]

'My first week back, I was only working one day a week, and I was absolutely shattered. I could have fallen asleep on my feet. And this was like six months afterwards. So I felt as though I ought to be getting stronger and quicker. And then I had about three months of relapse when I didn't do anything. I didn't do any keep-fit, or any walking. I just had a rest.'

I SUPPOSE PERCEPTION IS REALITY

'You don't realise—I suppose perception is reality—and you don't perceive how people see you. Like, I had a lot of friends in work that I didn't realise I had. A lot of people used to phone up. A lad at work used to come and pick me up: he used to park his car in the village, walk up and we'd walk down and have a cup of tea so I'd only have to walk one way. And it just touches you 'cos you think to yourself, "Oh, people don't care." But people do care; the only trouble is sometimes we perceive it as though they don't 'cos people ain't asking you every five minutes how you are. But once you've had like a major illness, people think, "Oh, bloody hell." Then it's like different. It just puts everything into perspective; it has for me.'

In negotiating the transition or 'rites of passage' between sickness and a return to some kind of normality, Jim feels aware of difference in himself, and in his relationships.

'I think most probably I'm a nicer person—if that's the right terminology.'

'So in what sense would you say nicer—how has that changed?' I ask him.

'I think with work colleagues and people I play golf with—I think I'm a little bit more dear to, whereas I always used to be like, not nasty, but everything had its place; work was work, golf was golf, or drinkin' with the boys on Friday night. I'd always think, "Why does he want to spend time with me?"'

'And now would you accept it more easily would you say?'

'Well perhaps I'm nicer—I always used to put barriers up. I didn't want people coming too close, like I didn't feel comfortable … I like people to stay … like over there. I'd say I'm closer to people; like a guy at work used to phone up every day, and say, "How you keeping, y'old bugger? Do you need anything?" I was thinking, bloody hell, we had a row six weeks ago and I was really rude to him, but then when you look back that's how we are. It's all about passion at that time.

'I think I move on a lot quicker, whereas before I'd think, "Oh he said something not very nice to me." I think to meself, well when I was ill, I was really touched by the amount of people that phoned up and sent cards, or popped into see me. In work they had a collection. One of them said, "I'm going out to see Jim. Anybody want to chuck a couple of quid in?" He said the word just spread. He said he was maybe thinking of getting like a magazine and a box of chocolates. But everybody was like, "Oh you're going to see Jim." And in the end he said, "We had to buy you five or six books." They … got me biographies, Colin Montgomery's, Alex Ferguson's, and it was touching. And so I try to put some of that back in; I try to think outside the box now. I know how good I felt, and now I try to listen a bit more and maybe look for a reason. Like in my job I need to discipline people; but I always try to look now for the reason why, what problems have they got. It might be a cry for help. Whereas before I'd be, "You done this; that is the punishment." I wouldn't even have lost a bit of sleep over it. But now I'm thinking a bit deeper about it and I think to meself how I would have felt.'

In reflecting on his own experience Jim is more able to imagine himself into the position of others:

'I think I'm a little bit more patient. Before, I wouldn't bend … whereas now, I will listen. What I gotta be careful of now, though … I don't want to get the reputation of Mr Softie who won't attack the issues, and I still feel that in my job I need to attack the issues. But you know, sometimes you can be a bit compassionate.

'There was a lad who 'ad a massive heart attack—I was there, and it was frightening as hell, 'cos I thought we'd actually lost 'im. And if it wasn't for the paramedics that was working on 'im … they done a fantastic job. But I'm a little bit more thoughtful—I try to remember how I felt. Like we do home visits, and we went to his flat and I was thinking that's how people live. And he'd got nobody; he'd got two daughters but his wife's buggered off and left him, and he's got kidney problems and heart problems. And I think he got more than enough to deal with without me puttin' me size nines all over his life.

'So he's coming back to work the next couple of weeks—and I know the barrier of coming through the door. Nobody else don't realise that barrier because they've never been there, but I have. I remember coming through those big green doors and thinkin' I don't want to go through there. I said to him, "You need to come back in and see me. I'll meet you in the car park and we can walk in together". 'Cos I can remember that's how it was.'

He draws on his own experience of going over the threshold of 'those big green doors' to support his colleague in making that transition. In finding meaning in his own experience, he is able to 'put some of that back in'.

TINS OF BEANS

'So I'm very pleased with that side of me life—I think I'm a little bit more understanding. I don't get angry as quick as I used to. And about life in general—I try to keep everything in its place. I used to really worry about work, but now I'm thinking, 'tins of beans'. I went to a meeting about 10 years ago, this guy said, "All we do is tins of beans; in the door, out the door—all we do is tins of beans". And I thought, "Isn't 'e ever right?" We all get so passionate about these tins of beans, but what does it matter if they don't get their tins of beans today, they can have 'em tomorrow. I think that was a massive lesson for me to learn. And after I 'ad me heart problems I just used to say it over in me mind, "tins of beans, in the door, out the door". And if you think about it, life's like that.'

The metaphor 'tins of beans' which is drawn from Jim's workplace acts as a useful analogy for his perspective on life.

'And it's about getting that perspective on life,' he adds. 'I mean, I've had two cracking shifts the last two days. I got my appraisal Tuesday morning. Now, say two years ago, I'd be absolutely terrified. I'd be thinking, "What if he says, you haven't done this or you haven't done that?" I don't care. He can say what he likes and I'll just say to him, "Yeah, alright." And I found that I'm saying that more and more. I'm thinking to myself, I don't need to go there. I don't need to get angry. But I think also I celebrate success more as well.'

'In what way, would you say?' I ask.

'In every way. I don't know if that's because of having the near-death experience or having a life-threatening experience, but I do celebrate success much more. If we've had a good shift in work, now I'll make a point of saying, "We had a cracking shift today," and I get the meal vouchers out—and I say, "Fantastic shift today, well done, boys".'

YOU CAN'T EXPLAIN THAT

I ask Jim more about the ways in which the experience has changed his attitude to life and death.

'It's hard to explain to people. No one will ever understand how it feels when you've been to the wall, and what I mean by that is when you close your eyes and go to sleep not knowing if you're going to wake up—you can't explain that to anybody.'

'No, you can't.'

'But you must recognise that,' he says to me, 'whereas someone who's never ever been there … I didn't sleep well for ages, and I'm talking like a long time afterwards. I used to sleep for a couple of hours then wake up. I might not go to sleep for another couple of hours. People just don't know and never understand how that feels, how you live with that.'

Paradoxically in that moment of expressing the loneliness of 'no-one will ever understand', Jim is able to acknowledge that I also 'must recognise that feeling', and that alongside the isolation of illness, there is common humanity. When we experience life-threatening illness we are divided from, but also united in, that most universal and existential of human conditions.

'You know, lying down and closing your eyes and not knowing if you're going to wake up or if you would ever wake up …'

'So it leaves you with a sense of awareness of all that, and fear …?' I ask him.

'Yes, definite fear … and after a bit you think, well I can't do anything about that anyway. What can I do? Nothing … if I'm gonna go, I'm gonna go … so that took a bit of getting me head round, which the counsellor helped me with.'

'And has it changed your attitude to life?' I ask him.

'It must have changed, because it's a life-changing thing. I can't say, put my hand on my heart—excuse the pun!—that it's changed. I love my house. I love my wife. I love my family. I did before—maybe not as much as now. I think like, once you've been to that wall, everything becomes different, everything becomes a first, everything feels … like going abroad for the first time, going for long car drives, journeys or anything.

HOPEFULLY I'LL MAKE OLD BONES

'You get to a stage where you think, I could sit in this chair and wait for God to come along, or I could get on with my life, and the decision we made was we'll carry on but be sensible whenever we can. And as long as you do that, as long as you don't have burger and chips every day, you don't have 10 pints of cider or a curry every day. Hopefully I'll make old bones. And there's no reason I shouldn't—I mean, we eat healthy, I go to the gym three times a week, play golf a couple of times a week when possible.'

'So would you say you do those things much more so now than you did before your heart attack?' I ask.

'Yes, definitely … much more. And I'm more mindful of what I'm eating. I go through bad stages as we all do, chocolate cakes, but I try to be a little bit more sensible if I can—which is difficult sometimes. Like whenever I go to a meeting at work there will always be chocolate and cakes as rewards for achievement—it's part of that supermarket culture; if someone does well, everyone has a slice of cake—nice, gooey chocolate cake. You can't go, "No I don't want that". But my daughter's getting married, and I want to lose some weight. So that's motivation to keep healthy as well. I've got into the gym in a big way in the last six months or so.'

'And it sounds like you're very committed to doing that, and it's a goal that you're working towards,' I reflect.

'But it's hard to explain to people, they don't understand if you miss one day then you sort of go back a day, it becomes harder. I'm quite regimented when I get to the gym. I have twenty minutes on the bike, and then I'll do five minutes rowing, then I'll do four minutes walking.'

'So you've got a real system,' I comment.

'Yes, and you mucked that system up; today I could only do 10 minutes!' he laughs. 'But only for today. It's alright, 'cos I'll go back tomorrow. Then Friday I'll either play golf or I'll go to the gym and if I can do like an hour every day.'

Laughing, I ask, 'So were you quite systematic before you were ill?'

'I've always been 100 per cent, whatever I do. I used to do lists, and of course I'm Mr Organised—10 minutes on the bike; five on the rower; 10 on the stepper, and I'd be running for four minutes. And I like to do it in that order as well.'

'So what's that about then?' I wonder.

'I don't know … if I do that, I feel as though it's completed, it's alright. I feel as though I'm getting fitter … the left side here is a bit twitchy; it's like a muscle I haven't used. It's just starting to come back again, so that worries me. When it's happening I think, Oh is that indigestion, or is it …? I mean, this morning I felt awful going out. But once I was there, the golf was on the telly and I was wired up, and I was thinking, "Oh isn't this nice?" I could have stayed there all day; it does give me a little sense of security. So touch wood, I've been keeping really well. And Louise works in a clinic, so if there is anything, she can ask the nurses. Our surgery's pretty good as well; I can just go down any morning.'

I ask how conscious Jim was of fitness before his heart attack, which leads him to reflect on how he accounts for it.

'Yeah, a little bit, a little bike ride, walking and golf. Most probably I drank and ate a bit too much … and a little bit hereditary, 'cos my parents had heart problems. I think I was under a bit of pressure at work. And that was why I was eating and drinking too much. I think it was those four things. Stress at work, being overweight, eating and drinking too much and hereditary. So it was all in place and they started to work in tandem. But I still didn't see it coming.'

'Yeah, I remember one of the phrases you used—you said you had that feeling that you were bulletproof, and then suddenly …'

'You're not,' he responds.

'I'm thinking of the way in which illness can change the directions of people's lives, and I'm wondering: have you experienced, like a sense of loss? There are things that we lose, but there can also be things that we gain. I wondered if you'd had any thoughts about that?' I ask him.

'I don't think I've lost anything really—I've always been happy with my lot. I had a nice life before, and I got a nice life afterwards. This is just like a little test along the way, I s'pose. And I come through that test and out the other side. But I went through stages. I was frustrated that I was earning good money and the house was all paid for and we got a few quid in our pockets. But I got back into my golf, which was really good … in fact better, 'cos my handicap's lower now!'

'Right!' I laugh.

He looks reflective. 'It's like a distant memory now. Although it was only a few years ago, it seems distant … and even today I look in the mirror thinking, "What's that?" looking at the scar …'

The fear and uncertainty are there for Jim, but he keeps them at bay, and by striving to keep fit and to eat more healthily has found a way of keeping them in the background and of living his life.

I ask him what he wants to result from his part in this research, or if there is any message he would like to convey.

'I think if it can help somebody, then I feel maybe I'm putting something back.

'And the message has got to be,' he continues, 'no matter what happens, you've got to make that conscious decision of where you want to go; the decision for me was when I sat there not long after my operation thinking, I don't like this. I need to be getting my life back. I felt as though someone was trying to cheat me out of my life, and I wanted to get back playing golf, get back fitness, and just enjoy me life a little bit more. I think I made a conscious decision of: no I'm not gonna sit and wait for God. No. I'm gonna get on. And I think the message is although we're all made up the same—two eyes, nose, mouth and ears—we're all different. Inside we're all different, and so complicated.'

Jim had found his own particular way of accommodating the freedom and the anxiety of life-threatening illness, and in doing so had turned, in Frank's[22] terms, the 'chaos' and 'restitution' stories into one of 'quest'. In making meaning and engaging in a transformative process, he was singing his own 'Song of Freedom'.

REFERENCES

1. Kendall M. Poems from the heart: living with heart failure. In: Hurwitz B, Greenhalgh T, Skultans V, editors. *Narrative Research in Health and Illness*. London: BMJ Books; 2004.
2. Clandinin J, Connelly FM. *Narrative Inquiry: experience and story in qualitative research*. San Francisco: Jossey-Bass; 2000.
3. Holroyd G. Men's health in perspective. In: Jones L, Sidell M, editors. *The Challenge of Promoting Health: exploration and action*. Buckingham, UK: Open University Press; 1997. pp. 209–18.
4. McVittie C, Willock J. You can't fight windmills: how older men do health, ill health, and masculinities. *Qualitative Health Research*. 2006; **16**(6): 788–801.
5. Clandinin, Connelly, op cit.
6. Bruner J. *Making Stories: law, literature, life*. New York: Farrar, Straus and Giroux; 2002.
7. BBC Television. *Dr. Who* [television programme]. 1963–present.
8. Frank A. *The Wounded Storyteller: body, illness and ethics*. Chicago, IL: University of Chicago Press; 1995.
9. Bruner J. Narratives of Plight: A conversation with Jerome Bruner. In: Charon R, Montello M. *Stories Matter: the role of narrative in medical ethics*. New York, NY: Routledge; 2002b.
10. Ricoeur, P. (1983) *Time and Narrative*. Chicago, IL: University of Chicago Press.
11. Sacks O. *A Leg to Stand On*. Revised Edition, London: Picador; 1991.
12. Bowlby J. *Attachment and Loss: separation, anxiety and anger (Vol.2)*. New York: Basic Books; 1973.
13. Becker G. *Disrupted Lives: how people create meaning in a chaotic world*. Berkeley and Los Angeles, CA: University of California Press; 1999.
14. Marley B. Redemption Song. *Uprising* [recording]. Island; 1980.
15. Sacks, op cit.
16. Martin V. *Out of my Head*. Lewes: Book Guild; 1997.
17. Griffiths P. Counselling in rehabilitation: the UK story. In: Etherington K, editor. *Rehabilitation Counselling in Physical and Mental Health*. London: Jessica Kingsley; 2002.
18. Etherington K, editor. *Rehabilitation Counselling in Physical and Mental Health*. London: Jessica Kingsley; 2002.
19. Hession J. At the Heart of Change: the impact of cardiac surgery on men's lives [unpublished MSc thesis]. University of Bristol; 2003.
20. Turner V. *The Ritual Process: structure and anti-structure*. Ithaca, NY: Cornell University Press; 1969.
21. Van Gennep A. *The Rites of Passage*. London: Routledge and Kegan Paul; 1960.
22. Frank, op cit.

CHAPTER 5

Yasmin's story

INTRODUCTION

Yasmin is in her 40s and has had Crohn's disease, a form of inflammatory bowel disease (IBD), for 15 years.[1,2] She has had many bowel operations, including a temporary colostomy and a permanent ileostomy. The siting of the ileostomy has been problematic; high output and consistency of waste through the stoma (the opening in the body where the bag is fitted) has meant that it is very difficult to manage. The nature of Yasmin's condition is unpredictable: the bag needs emptying frequently and therefore she has a loss of control over getting rid of waste. Her illness affects her whole body system; it unbalances her body chemistry and causes dehydration. She has had serious infections including peritonitis and septicaemia and has been in intensive care on several occasions. She has to have blood tests every week, and has needed frequent hospitalisation to the degree that this illness has taken over her life and disrupted most of what was her previous life.

Severe IBD can have a profound and long-term impact on the quality of life and sense of self and identity of the individual. It is, as Thomas[3] writes, 'at best an extremely unpleasant disease to live with and can, at worst, be devastating' (p. 132). 'The symptoms which fluctuate unpredictably, can give rise to much anguish, embarrassment and shame' (p. 133). The silence and shame that surround IBD mean that the voices of sufferers are seldom heard, making it a particularly isolating disease; therefore there is a great need for counselling support which offers the time and space in which to tell the stories of how it is to live with the devastation that this condition can cause.[4,5]

I was put in touch with Yasmin through a colleague in the counselling field. As someone with severe inflammatory bowel disease that had necessitated surgery, she had experienced a profound and long-term assault on her sense of self and life story. Yasmin's story exemplifies, as clearly as any story can, the rupture to the sense of self and life course following the devastation of serious illness. 'Order' as Becker[6] writes, 'begins with the body' (p. 12). When that body, whose 'taken-for-granted-ness' can no longer be taken for granted, is thrown into chaos and disorder, the present and the future are replete with uncertainty. Her story is, as Bruner[7] puts it, 'deeply about plight, about the road rather than about the inn to which it leads' (p. 20). For Yasmin, the road goes ever on; it is a lonely road and one that powerfully illustrates the existential isolation of illness.

While I am acutely aware that I can never fully convey the relentless present and bleak future of Yasmin's illness, which took away hope and confined life, I will try and take the reader into her world as she unfolded it with me. Yasmin's life has been characterised by unremitting suffering, acute drama, and an abiding 'deep and nameless sadness' (p. 17) for the last 15 years.[8] She has lived continuously in the abyss of her illness.

Charon[9] writes of the storytelling process as a 'dance of confirmation', a reciprocal exchange in which 'participants are gravely and joyously giving and receiving at the same time' (p. 60). That is indeed my hope; but I am aware that any joy for Yasmin has long since departed, and the story she tells shows little promise of transformation, or change for the better. All I can offer is my commitment to active and respectful listening, and to bearing witness to her story.

IT HAS CHANGED WHO I AM … CHANGED MY LIFE

I step from the train and see a woman on her own looking round for someone. I tentatively walk towards her as she looks up and sees me approaching.

'Hi. Are you Yasmin?' I enquire as she says in the same instant, 'Viv?'

We shake hands and smile. 'The car's just through here,' she says as she leads me out of the station. 'I live very close.' We arrive a few minutes later at her home, a modern flat close to the station.

We sit with coffee, and I go through the initial contracting information: details of confidentiality, anonymity and so on. I know how important it is to discuss these issues, yet I want to 'get these things out of the way' so that I can hear her story uninterrupted. And I sense that for Yasmin, this is also the case.

She asks me, 'So, what are you actually looking for in this research? '

I tell her briefly what has led me into this project, and then say, 'What I'm interested in is what it's like to live with the kind of condition that you have and the impact of that on your life and your sense of who you are—that sense of identity and the way in which serious illness sends lives in directions that we could not have imagined … in a nutshell, that's what it's about. How do you feel about that?' I ask. 'Do you have any feeling about whether taking part in this might be for you?'

'Definitely,' she says emphatically. 'I've definitely been affected by it, my whole life. It has changed who I am …changed my personality … changed my life.'

'So if you were to tell me your story from the beginning, how would you start?' I ask her.

'I would start about 15 years ago. For a couple of weeks I had quite a bad tummy pain, sickness, and diarrhoea. I kept ignoring it, going to work … I was a single parent, taking Jenny to nursery. I was going to work full time and ignoring it. And then one night, it was horrendously bad. I managed to take Jen to nursery next morning and then went to my doctor's surgery. I walked in the door and passed out … next thing I knew I was in the ambulance. They thought that my appendix had ruptured, so they whisked me off to hospital. People in the hospital agreed that it was my appendix. That afternoon they took me down to surgery. When they got there, my appendix looked fine but they took it out anyway, looked a bit further, and that's when they could see that my bowel was inflamed and swollen. Then they took a biopsy. They said it could be Crohn's or colitis; if it was Crohn's, that could be treated with drugs. If it was colitis, I would need further surgery.'

She takes a sip of coffee, and continues. 'I came home. I was still being sick, I had diarrhoea. When the biopsy results came back two weeks later, they showed Crohn's and I was put on steroids for maybe 10 weeks ...'

She pauses. 'They never helped. I'd take the steroids, but the only time they worked was if I'd go into hospital and have them intravenously. Then within two days it would be back to normal and it was great. I'd come home, go back to work, and everything would be fine. And then within a week I'd be back on tablets and would start to go down again. When I first became ill, I lost a lot of weight. But once I was on steroids, I gained enormously. I went from ten stone to fourteen stone in months. And that had such an effect on me, just putting on weight. I would have times when I would be quite well. And then I'd be ill, and I'd lose weight. They'd give me steroids and I'd put on weight.'

There are questions I want to ask, but I know this is not the time. The story is waiting to be told, and *will* be told. It pours out—a catalogue of events and experiences. There will be time, I know, in later conversations, when her experiences will be examined in fine and harrowing detail; there will be times when meanings will emerge; and times when words will not be enough to express the profound sadness that illness has brought to Yasmin's life. For the present, I silently receive the gift of Yasmin's story.

'After about a year of being in and out of hospital, of having intravenous steroids and trying to cope with steroids at home, they decided that they were going to remove the diseased bit of bowel. They would cut a piece out and then rejoin the bowel, stitch it together and I'd be fine. So I went in, had the operation and I was fine for probably six months.

'It went on like that for five years, and every year I'd end up going into hospital and they'd cut a little bit of bowel out and I'd be fine for six months. Then the process would start again.'

At the same time as being a single mother with responsibility for a young child, and a house to maintain, Yasmin worked full-time. But somehow she managed to cope with all of that and provide a secure, loving home for her daughter.

THAT'S IT ... MY LIFE'S OVER

'After about five years I went in to have another bit removed, and that's when it really changed ... looking back on it, the first five years were quite good, really,' she says, without a hint of irony. 'Compared to what happened next ...'

She pauses. 'I went back in to have it removed. Everything was fine, and about four days after the operation I started to get quite poorly; it started swelling up. I was having trouble breathing. Apparently what had happened was, where they had rejoined the bowel, the stitching had broken down; so all the contents of my bowel had leaked into my body and got onto my lungs. Both my lungs collapsed and I had peritonitis and septicaemia. I was just… well, three weeks of my life—I just lost. I have no recollection of that at all. People have told me since, obviously. They did a temporary colostomy.

'I remember waking up and I had this bag stuck onto my stomach and obviously I was aware of colostomies, but I thought it was something that would happen when I was 70. Not in my 30s. I can remember saying to my sister at the time … I looked at her, and I said, "That's it, my life's over, how am I going to live with a bag stuck to my stomach?" They said, "Oh, it's only temporary, and it'll be alright." I was in hospital that time for about three months with an open wound, the size of a fist. I had MRSA (Methicillin-resistant Staphylococcus aureus). I had fistulas. At one point, I had three bags on my tummy collecting different fluids from my body. I wasn't allowed on the ward. I wasn't allowed to use the bathroom, I had this tiny, tiny room where I slept, ate, went to the toilet, washed …'

I know something of the loneliness of serious illness, but this … this separation from life, even from hospital life, such as it is. This, I can barely imagine. My next words echo my inadequacy in the face of such desolation: 'So you were really isolated?'

'To me, that was really the beginning of it completely changing my life. I just felt, I don't know … it was like, if anyone came in to see me, they had to wear gloves and aprons. And I just felt so isolated. I remember one time I went out to buy a paper from the little trolley thing and this nurse said, "You're not allowed out of your room." I couldn't talk to any other patients. That was a hard time, and I just thought, I'm never going to get better—but though I say I did, I've never got back to how I was.'

How I *was*: the before and after of sickness; the self whose fragile body stumbles, then falls. How difficult just to keep going; to have no choice *but* to keep going. I gravely attend to her continuing story.

'But I was well enough to come home and get on with things,' she continues. 'Then about a year later, I went back in and had the colostomy reversed. Again, it didn't work. The stitching broke down and everything leaked. I was back in intensive care. I had a tracheotomy; I couldn't breathe on my own, I was hooked up to machines. I don't remember it, but apparently they called my family in twice because they thought my time was very limited.

'They kept saying to me I need you to have an ileostomy, and it would be permanent. And I didn't want it. I just couldn't. It was hard enough with the colostomy, knowing that was temporary, but knowing that this would be for the rest of my life … I didn't want it, and I kept saying no, I don't want it. If I'm poorly, I'm poorly. My surgeon eventually had very stern words with me and said he couldn't guarantee how long I'd last if I didn't have the operation. Then obviously I had it. I would like to have said I had it and everything was fine afterwards. But they did this ileostomy and again I was in intensive care for a few weeks, in hospital for three or four months and came home.'

I WAS LIKE A RECLUSE

'When I first I had the ileostomy, I had terrible leaks; I wouldn't go out because it would just leak all the time. I'd be in Sainsbury's, and it would leak … I remember once going out to dinner with Jenny; the waiter had just brought our food over and my bag leaked; we just had to get up and go. So, I was like a recluse. I couldn't go out anywhere.'

'So that sense of being part of the world was just taken away?' I say.

'It was just gone, completely gone. I couldn't keep my house anymore … it got to the stage where I was spending 24 hours in my bedroom. I didn't have a downstairs bathroom, and I couldn't walk up and down stairs. So I moved the kettle into my bedroom and I lived in my bedroom really and it was just awful, absolutely awful.'

Repeated admission to hospital meant that Yasmin was regularly separated from her daughter.

'It was awful for Jenny as well … she was just six when I was first diagnosed … and being a single parent, every time I went into hospital it was like, "Where's Jenny gonna go?" Her dad's around, but not reliably around. Many a time she'd go off to school in the morning and come home in the afternoon and I was in hospital. And I'd have to ring and say I've spoken to so and so, they'll come and pick you up.'

My heart goes out to this mother and her child. 'How hard for you …' I say.

'It was awful, 'cos I … the trouble is, I would leave it until I was so ill because I kept thinking I'll be fine tomorrow, and I didn't want to disrupt Jenny again. And I'd leave it till they had to carry me out on a stretcher.'

'You'd be kind of resisting it?' I ask with an empathy born of recognition.

'Absolutely … totally …'

The siting of the stoma has been problematic and has twice needed to be moved. The skin around the stoma is often very sore and can become infected. In addition, the volume and consistency of waste have meant that it is very difficult to manage: the bag needs emptying frequently, and therefore she has lost control over getting rid of waste, making her condition particularly isolating.

The chasm of sickness separates Yasmin from her previous self. Trapped in a relentless cycle of suffering, confined to her house, to her bedroom, to drips for nutrition, for rehydration, Yasmin was unable to return to work to the job she loved and the active social life she had once enjoyed. This severance from the person she had been affects every dimension of her life.

'Before all this, I used to be such an outgoing person. I was bubbly, sporty, energetic. I did two jobs. I was a single parent. I used to play badminton, swim, go to the gym. I rarely sat down, and two years before I became ill I'd moved into this house. We'd have people round, I was popular, I had a good life; a normal life. People would say, "Oh do you want to do something?" I didn't even think about it ... "Yeah I'll be there," I'd say ... the life and soul. I used to enjoy going to work. I was an accountant. I had a good job, I'd been promoted, and life was good.

'I haven't had a boyfriend for years now. I feel demoted. I'm very ashamed of my body. Very ashamed. I've got bags stuck here, and I've got scars. I've got me needle thing stuck up here. There's been a few times when I've been approached by men, but I just think I don't want the hassle of having to explain to them. I would hate having a boyfriend, to get involved with someone and then for them to see my bag and to be revolted by it. It would be awful, and I'd just rather not take the chance. But that's not me. Before I would have taken the chance whatever it was. It's been a long, long time, and I've accepted it ... but I don't know if I really have.'

As Kelly[10] writes, 'The ileostomy carries a freight of more or less socially signifi-cant symbols associated with dirt, pollution, loss of control and transgression of body margins' (p. 391). For Yasmin, the boundary between the private, personal, embodied self and the social self is transgressed whenever the bag leaks—as it does frequently. And thought of sexual intimacy is, as Thomas[11] notes, 'extraordinarily daunting, especially where a stable relationship has not yet been formed' (p. 134).

The profound alteration in body-image affects the most intimate and private domains of Yasmin's life; the need for connection with another, for partnership, intimacy and love are made so difficult as to be almost out of reach.

Yasmin's story epitomises the 'chaos narrative' whose 'plot imagines life never getting better'[12] (p. 97); for Yasmin, this is not just a temporary state, but a life lived in the midst of chaos. 'I said I would never let this illness control my life,' she tells me, 'but it's such an ongoing thing. This is how I've got to live. I don't want to live like this. But what can I do about it? I can't change it; I know this time next year it's gonna be the same.'

Yasmin lives with the contingency of illness all the time, in an unceasing present where hope has long departed and is ultimately and absolutely out of reach. Any brief respite is lived on the edge of this chaos.

ISOLATION

Yasmin's isolation within the medical setting is exemplified and also symbolised by the physical isolation she has to endure due to MRSA. But it is also marked in the sense that medicine does not offer what Frank refers to as the kind of 'restitution' that it promises. Her condition cannot easily be managed and certainly not 'cured'. As Frank[13] writes, 'Contemporary culture treats health as the normal condition that people ought to have restored. Thus the ill person's own desire for restitution is compounded by the expectation that other people want to hear restitution stories' (p. 77). The dominance of the 'restitution' storyline in Western culture thus models and constrains the stories that can be told. Frank notes, 'Chaos stories are as anxiety provoking as restitution stories are preferred' (p. 97). Where there is no clear trajectory of diagnosis, treatment and cure, then the person inhabiting the 'chaos story' suffers a lonely succession of events without meaning. Thomas, a specialist counsellor within a large gastroenterology unit, found that her clients 'felt that few people are able or willing to try to understand how they felt and believed that this was because their distress was too powerful and thus too painful for others to bear'[14] (p. 138).

Yasmin tells of repeated admissions to hospital. Again and again: for severe dehydration, near kidney failure, infections that take her to the edge of death.

I'M A PERSON TOO

She describes how her body is now so used to these chemical imbalances. 'I used to know. I'd start getting dizzy spells; I'd feel exhausted; my legs would feel like they didn't belong to me. But I don't know anymore. So I just keep going. The doctors say, "I cannot understand how you're standing, 'cos with these results here you should be almost comatose."

'When I have my bloods done, there are certain things that are always wrong, but now the doctors say, "Oh yes, for Yasmin that's fine." And I'm thinking to myself, I'm a person too. If it's not OK for you, then it shouldn't be for me. So it's almost like they've re-written their parameters,' she reflects. 'And it feels horrible. I say to them, "Why is it happening to me?" And they say, "We don't know … 'cos you're different … 'cos you're special." I don't want to be different and special. I just want them to get me better, you know? But they can't, and last time I was in hospital I was there for three weeks and they did nothing, 'cos there's nothing they *can* do.'

Her illness involves frequent and often emergency admission to hospital, where she would not usually see doctors who were familiar with the complex and long-term nature of her particular illness experience, nor have immediate access to her notes. This meant that at times the onus was on Yasmin to explain, for example, the significance of her blood results to an emergency on-call doctor.

'There was one time when my GP got my blood results and got me into hospital and my consultant said, "Yes it is low, but for you it's not too bad, and I don't think you need to stay here," and so I came home again, and from that point my GP said, "I can't be involved in this anymore, 'cos you're so specialised now that when I look at your blood results I interpret them as for a normal person." And from that point he didn't want my blood results anymore.'

Because Yasmin's experience does not follow the meta-narrative of diagnosis, treatment and cure, at times she feels abandoned by medicine. The long-term and ongoing suffering she endures has no place within the culturally preferred narrative of getting well. As Frank[15] points out, in a critique of the modernist narrative of the 'sick role', 'medical sympathy is to be limited by the overriding message that the sick person's task is to get well'[16] (p. 82).

'When I think of all the stuff they can do … they can give somebody a new heart, for God's sake. And yet they can't put me right. There may be medical advances—but the way things stand at the moment, I'm not gonna get better; it's only gonna get worse.'

Advances in medical science raise hopes and expectations which throw Yasmin's suffering into sharp relief and highlight her sense of despair and hopelessness.

'Is it as if the promise of medical science offers you nothing … you feel let down by it?' I ask.

'I *do* feel let down, *so* let down, and I just feel sometimes that medically now they can do so much, so why can't they do something for me? Do you know what I mean? There was this programme about face transplants, and I was thinking, how can they do that but not be able to do anything for me? Not even to give me a 20 per cent better life. I just want to be able to have some sort of a life, so I can go out socially; I haven't done that for such a long time. Or go on holiday.'

There are times when Yasmin feels abandoned by some doctors, and times when she feels things could have been done differently. Her feelings of desertion and isolation partly reside in the long-term, ongoing nature of her condition, and also in her sense that it is a condition which lacks the public profile and status of an illness such as cancer:

'With me and my illness—it's not something that I went through and then came out the other side. I'm still living it, and I've lived it for such a long time, and … it just seems so pointless really. Sometimes I think to myself, I wish I had cancer, 'cos if I had cancer there'd be a lot more help available, and people recognise it, and immediately people are sympathetic—they understand a little bit about it.'

Because Yasmin's condition is relatively invisible, her suffering is also invisible and can go unrecognised. As she points out, 'If someone's got a broken leg, they've got the plaster on and immediately people are sympathetic; there is some kind of understanding. Whereas for me … I mean I can't understand it, the doctors don't understand it … so how anyone else does … what they make of it.'

A visible 'sign', such as a plaster, which signifies a recognisable and well-known injury, arouses a sympathetic response, and also a degree of understanding, whereas the suffering caused by Yasmin's illness is relatively hidden, and not widely recognised or understood. The stigma of a bowel disease with its associations of bodily waste further compounds her sense of isolation.

Stories such as Yasmin's are neither easy to tell, nor to hear. There are few culturally available narratives representing IBD in the way that stories of, for example, cancer are available in the media. Such an intractable and relentless condition does not 'fit' the preferred 'getting back to normal' or 'fighting' models of illness and confounds everyone involved in her care, leaving her feeling abandoned at times; alone in a wilderness from which there is no escape, and where hope is out of reach.

I HAVEN'T GOT THAT HOPE ANY LONGER

'It just goes on and on and—when it was first diagnosed as Crohn's disease, there was always, "There'll be the operation and you'll be fine", and, "We'll do this and that will work out", or "We'll put you on steroids and that will bring it under control." There was always a hope. Do you know what I mean? And I haven't got that hope any longer ... I suppose I just have to accept my lot; they're not gonna make it better at the moment. I just feel so downtrodden by it. When I first see a new doctor, they're all like: "I'm gonna get you better", and then one by one they try and it doesn't work and I feel that they've written me off ... what they've expected to work hasn't worked, and every single time each doctor I've had has given up.'

'And what do you think that's about? Do you think that's at a human level, or built into the system?' I ask.

'I can see—especially with my doctor now—how frustrated he is, 'cos he can't make me better. And it's almost like he feels he's failed with me, but he doesn't want to admit he's failed. But he doesn't actually do anything. I think to be honest that there are too many demands now. And I almost feel I'm ignored, 'cos the conventional things haven't worked. I never see my consultant unless it's an emergency. It'll just be the next time I have a problem, I'll get rushed in and I'll see him.'

What Yasmin is asking for is healing; it is almost as if she is saying, 'If cure is not possible, then at least don't turn away. Recognise me. Stand with me in my pain and feel for my spirit. Even if you can't treat me, then care for me. I am not "other". I am a fellow human being. Offer me your fellowship and humanity.' She asks for an empathy born of human connection and the willingness, delicacy and courage to enter her 'private perceptual world'[17] (p. 142) and to dwell there however temporarily, bearing witness to her suffering. When cure is not possible, then perhaps all we can hope for or offer is *presence*.

At times, she is stuck in a limbo between hospital and home, with the ambiguous status of being well enough to be discharged but not well enough to live her life. The relentless nature of her illness leaves her in a netherworld where she is temporarily, and usually fleetingly, free from hospitalisation, though never from patienthood. She inhabits a limbo in which she cannot, and dare not, belong to the outside world, for she knows that such belonging will be snatched from her:

'Sometimes I wish I didn't have the good bits. 'Cos it only feels worse when it all goes again. It's like one step forward, and 10 steps back. It's so, so good—but then when it drops down, it's so, so bad. And then I think, *Why* do I bother? *What* is the point?'

Yasmin wants to resist illness, but also needs to be aware of shifts and changes in her body. I ask her, 'Does that leave you with a sense of responsibility for monitoring your own condition?'

'Yes, yes—which I'm not very good at, because I leave it too late. I leave it till I'm so, so poorly. I just think well, I'll see how I am tomorrow.'

'I remember you said last time, part of that is because you feel that they might judge you on it.'

'Yes, yes … and they do. My doctor said to me that he felt that I was becoming too comfortable with being in hospital—which is probably again why I leave it so long. I don't want people to feel sorry for me. I don't want people to think, "Oh, it's Yasmin—she's in hospital again, never mind, that's where she's happiest."'

'Like you don't want people to make any assumptions that this is your choice, 'cos it is *not*?' I ask.

'Yes. And I honestly think some doctors think that I'm choosing to be poorly. It makes me feel very uncomfortable. I just feel they've given up on me. And then I think to myself, Well what can they do? I don't know what they can do. I don't know … I sort of limp along from one crisis to the next, and when I have a crisis, I get rushed into hospital and they do whatever they do. Then I come home, and I limp along till the next one, but there's nothing in-between; they forget about me until the next crisis comes up …

'My doctor said to me about a year ago that he'd be quite happy if I wanted to get a second opinion, and I said, "I've had so many opinions, and each time I've gone to a new doctor, they've done all the same tests, tried the same things, then eventually come to the same conclusion." I've even been to a specialist hospital in London, and they came up with "don't know". And I'm fed up with "I don't knows". I said to him a while ago, "Whatever you say, do *not* say you don't know. I don't want to hear that anymore." *Why* don't they know? *Why* don't they know? The things they can do. *Why* is it so different for me? Why?'

I JUST HAD NO LIFE AT ALL

It is as if Yasmin is stuck in the middle of a story: an unrelenting story without understanding or explanation. She tells of the struggle to find hope in the face of isolation that has transformed her world into to one of pain, mess, and disgust; and her life into one of limitations, unpredictability, and continual struggle.

'It must be very hard to find something to look forward to, to find hope in a sense?' I say.

'I don't. If I hadn't had Jenny … well … about a year and a half ago, I took an overdose, 'cos I just felt I don't want to live. If it's gonna be like the last year, I'd rather not be around. That's what prompted them to do the stoma. I just had no life at all. I'd wake up at two o'clock in the morning and my bag would leak and I'd gotta get up, strip my bed, have a bath. Sometimes I just used to move to the other side of the bed. When I think about it now, I feel disgusted with myself.'

'Living with it sounds just so impossible,' I say.

'Yes … yes it is.'

'So how do you keep yourself going?' I ask in awe.

'Jenny. Basically, that's it. When she goes back to university, I look forward to the holidays. And I look forward to the phone call in the week. And when she's here she does help me. And I feel I have to get up and get dressed. When she's not here,

I could go a week in my pyjamas. I have times when I won't answer the phone. I don't want to say to someone, "I feel poorly again." I said that to them last time. And I can't lie, 'cos they're gonna know by my voice. So I don't answer the phone.'

She pauses. 'And I've got used to it. I don't like it, but I've sort of accepted it. I tried to do a little job at a charity shop just one afternoon a week. But I couldn't even do that, because I couldn't commit myself to the same times. That was just the pits—I couldn't even manage a couple of hours a week in a charity shop.'

'I imagine your whole sense of being part of the outside world …' I tentatively say.

'I'm *not* part of the outside world. Not anymore. Being in hospital for such a length of time sort of cocoons you. And then when you come out … I've had panic attacks in Sainsbury's, 'cos I'm not used to the noise and the amount of people. Everything's just too much.'

'I can remember coming out of hospital and finding the outside world quite overwhelming,' I say.

'It's a very scary place. And it's really difficult, 'cos I spend so much time in hospital. If I come out and got used to the outside world again it would be harder when I go back in. And in my mind, I know that my future is in and out of hospital, so I don't want to break that mould. Do you know what I mean?' she asks.

'Yes I do; is it like, if you adjust too fully to living in the outside world it's going to be harder going back in?' I ask.

'That's right; it's going to be really hard. And the way it's been, I've spent more time in hospital than I have out. So it's best if I'm in that frame of mind—which is an awful way to be.'

'That's a very hard way to live your life. I imagine it almost feels like you're not living your life; you're in this sort of half world,' I say.

'Yeah, I haven't lived my life for a long time. I always used to say I wasn't going to let Crohn's control my life. It was part of my life, I couldn't do anything about that, but that was it. But illness rules my life and it has to. I have to make sure that I've got the intravenous stuff. That takes 18 hours a day, so I've got to find 18 hours out of 24 when I can sit and have the intravenous nutrition (TPN) and the fluids. Even if I have one bag, that takes six hours; a big chunk of the day.'

'And how do you get through those periods? When you are having to stay in one place for six hours or for 18 hours?' I ask her.

'Sitting, looking out the window, I don't watch a lot of telly. I listen to music quite a bit. Sometimes I read, sometimes I don't. A lot of the time I just sit, I can't really do anything; I just sit and I feel sorry for myself I suppose. I *do* feel sorry for myself. I keep saying I shouldn't, but I do. It's so unfair. It's the way they can't put me right.'

When I next see Yasmin, we talk more about her attempted suicide. In the intervening two months she has spent yet more time in hospital through severe infection and dehydration. Her Hickman line, the catheter in her chest used for long-term intravenous access, had become severely infected, and had required surgery to remove it. The infection then spread into her blood stream. In addition, she had become seriously dehydrated and close to kidney failure.

WHEN IT'S YOUR TIME …

Tentatively I say, 'Can I ask—say if you don't want to talk about this—but you have been close to death on several occasions, and so you have lived and you continue to live with that … on the edge of that at times. Also, I know that there are times when you've felt "I don't know if I want to live" … I want to ask how it is for you to live with that? … I understand if you don't want to answer.'

'I do … I do.'

'And the other part of the question is how do you make sense of that in terms of your beliefs about life and death? And how do you place all that in the bigger picture?'

'I sort of have the philosophy that when it's your time, it's your time … and it's not been my time. I've been close lots of times really … and one time I even tried to make it happen, but over the years I've decided that when it's time for you to die you will die. It's like … when they said to me … there's a real chance you could die, I almost don't believe it anymore, 'cos I've been there before and it didn't happen … and there are other times when I think I wish I had died. They said to me, "You've been fighting", and I've thought why did I struggle just for this? But I do think that when it's your time it's your time, and you can't change that … and it just hasn't been my time yet.'

I ask, 'And the time when you did nearly make it happen, how do you make sense of that now? How was it at the time, and how do you see that looking back on it?'

'At the time I really felt that the life I had wasn't a life worth having, and not just for me, but for everybody around me. I felt that I'd had enough, and I still get times when I feel like that. I can remember waking up and being really disappointed that I'd woken up. And in my mind—and still today—I'd had a valid reason for doing what I did—it wasn't some whim. I had decided. I had made that choice, and for me it was a rational choice. It was something I'd thought about for a long time. I'd thought how I could do it, but then I woke up and obviously it was still not my time. And sometimes I wish it was, 'cos it would be over by now.'

'Can I ask … it sounds almost that part of you had really had enough, but there's another part—a spirit there—that keeps you going, and that kind of knows that it's not time?'

'Yes … I do firmly believe that from the moment you're born your time is already decided when you're gonna die, and it doesn't matter what you do, you can't avoid that. And I think, in a way, the times when I nearly died through illness and the time when I tried to make it happen and I didn't succeed made me believe it even more, you know? I have days when I think, gosh, I wish it was my time ... but I know it's not, and I know that I can't bring it forward. I know that I can't force it to happen. But I say to myself why isn't it my time? What life have I actually got? So why is it not my time? Almost why am I being made to suffer so much? I remember reading an article once which said that people suffer in their life because of the bad things they did in a previous life ... I don't believe it ... and I don't believe in God; I think if there was a god, how could he just stand by and see so much suffering.'

We talk about her fear that she would be judged as 'taking the easy way out', and of the aftermath of attempted suicide. We talk of how such stories cannot be easily told ... of the shame attached to stories of suicide, a shame that silences and isolates the storytellers.

I think of my own need to 'make sense of' and to create meaning from illness experience, and of how impossible a task it would be if I inhabited a sequence of events without form or ending as Yasmin does, always in the middle of this story. The isolation of serious illness is so powerful and real while we are in the middle of the experience and in some ways recedes when we re-enter the domain of the well. I no longer live with it in an everyday, all-day sense ... yet it is something I do remember, something I fear, something I am reminded of when I have health problems. It has been in the process of writing this that I have come to realise just how much of the hopelessness and search for meaning in relation to serious illness I have 'forgotten'. I have needed to consciously 'go there' in my mind and to dwell in it in order to reconnect with the chasm that is 'that deep and nameless sadness', and to access some of my own resonance with Yasmin's experience.

DO YOU CROSS THE BRIDGE?

I do not see Yasmin for nearly four months, most of which she has spent in hospital. Then one day I receive a joyous phone call.

'This last two weeks—honestly, Viv, it's like a miracle ... it was suddenly one day ... and you know I was in hospital for two-and-a-half months. It was an awful time, and I came home and I was quite well ... then about a week after coming home I had flu, and I got quite low, and then I started being sick. The doctor thought I might have an infection on my Hickman line, so he prescribed antibiotics. I took those and within about four days ...' She clicks her fingers. 'Suddenly—it wasn't gradual—it was, "I feel better."' Her voice radiates joy and hope.

When I see her, she sparkles with zest for life. There is a playfulness about her, but underlying her lightness of spirit is the fear and foreboding that this will not last. She is seizing life with both hands, but is also so afraid that this is but a temporary respite, a cruel glimpse of the life she would love, but cannot have: 'I could wake up tomorrow feeling poorly. And I'd go back down in a second,' she tells me.

She talks about songs that have resonance and meaning for her, and quotes from 'The Bridge' by Elton John:[18] 'It says, *Do you cross the bridge or do you fade away*'. Then she says, joy spilling from her, 'Two weeks ago I couldn't cross the bridge, and I was fading away. But now I've crossed the bridge.'

To my delight, she sends me a text the following week:

'Hi Viv, hope you're well. Things STILL good with me! I heard this song and the lyrics sum up how I've been feeling recently! Natasha Bedingfield—Unwritten. *Feel the rain on your face. No-one else can feel it for you. Today is where your book begins, the rest is still unwritten …!*[19] Have a listen! Take care x'

But three weeks later, I have a call to tell me that she is back in hospital with yet another infection. She has collapsed, and her system, which is so 'battered and undermined', has 'crashed'. She is critically ill, in intensive care and might not survive. Her close friend says to me, 'She may survive this, but how will she get through it?'

Yasmin does survive this collapse; she spends a month in hospital, and emerges from this critical stage very weak. She sends me a wonderful text message full of warmth and humour: 'Hi Viv, thank you so much for the card and your kind words. I am on the mend but still very weak. My goal at the moment is to get rid of the zimmer frame!! I hope everything is good with you and I'll try and ring you soon. Take care x'

We spoke after she was discharged from hospital. She said she was feeling 'loads better' but was afraid it wouldn't last: 'I could wake up tomorrow morning, and it's all gone to pot.'

She talks of a song by Cat Stevens:[20] '*Oh Very Young* came on the radio, and I stopped what I was doing, and I listened. He sings of the short while we dance on the earth, of how our dreams fade and vanish. And I thought this is such a powerful, meaningful song, and it means so much to me.'

And the ending of this story? Where? How does it end? Does it end? How do *I* end Yasmin's story in a way that conveys what Spence[21] terms the 'narrative truth' of her experience? For endings are constructs, fictional patterns we impose on experience. In the words of Frank Kermode, 'the end is like infinity plus one and imaginary numbers in mathematics, something we know does not exist but which help us to make sense of and to move in the world'[22] (p. 3). It seems to me that a fundamental feature of Yasmin's lived experience of illness, is that it *just goes on*; her story is without a clear or straightforward ending; it is ongoing, fraught with uncertainty, and inconclusive. She lives her story suspended in time.

As Mattingly[23] writes, 'Plot gives unity to an otherwise meaningless succession of one thing after another' (p. 46). For Yasmin, who frequently feels she is stuck in the middle of a story without an ending, this 'formlessness is not so much a description of the structure of everyday life as a depiction of despair. The essence of meaninglessness is when lived experience seems to be driven by no form other than brute sequence'[24] (p. 47). Her story highlights, in a most cruel and extreme way, what is true for any of us: that the struggle to find meaning and purpose and identity is fundamentally threatened by the contingencies of serious illness. Yasmin's experience of relentless suffering raises questions about what constitutes 'living', for as she said, 'At the time, I really felt that the life I had wasn't a life worth having.' Yalom[25] identifies four basic existential challenges in life: death, freedom, isolation and meaning. Yasmin's story seems to me to crystallise all of those challenges, and to bring them sharply and poignantly into focus.

POSTSCRIPT

Four months after I had written the previous section, Yasmin died. She was in hospital again, and her heart stopped. Resuscitation was attempted. But she died: with clarity, certainty and inevitability. Her death was unexpected though always anticipated. Her time had come.

In Pullman's *The Amber Spyglass*,[26] the guardians of the 'land of the dead' are given the task of asking 'every ghost to tell you the story of their lives' (p. 333). As I have been thinking and writing this postscript to Yasmin's illness story, I am reminded that every life-story is the story of a life. Yasmin's story is one of suffering and fear, of struggle for hope and search for meaning, of resilience alongside frailty, and of invincibility alongside immense vulnerability. There was a sparkle about Yasmin's spirit—I *really* liked her. I feel honoured to have known her—albeit briefly—and to have been given the privilege of working with her story.

REFERENCES

1. Thomas G. *Counselling and Reflexive Research in Healthcare: working therapeutically with clients with inflammatory bowel disease.* London: Jessica Kingsley; 2009.
2. Thomas G. Counselling people with ulcerative colitis. In: Etherington K, editor. *Rehabilitation Counselling in Physical and Mental Health.* London: Jessica Kingsley; 2002a. pp.131–45.
3. Ibid.
4. Thomas, 2009, op cit.
5. Kelly M. Self, identity and radical surgery. *Sociol Health Illn.* 1992; **14**(3): 390–415.
6. Becker G. *Disrupted Lives: how people create meaning in a chaotic world.* Berkeley and Los Angeles, CA: University of California Press; 1999.
7. Bruner J. *Making Stories: law, literature, life.* New York: Farrar, Straus and Giroux; 2002.
8. Charon R. *Narrative Medicine: honoring the stories of illness.* Oxford: Oxford University Press; 2006.
9. Ibid.
10. Kelly, op cit.
11. Thomas, 2002, op cit.
12. Frank A. *The Wounded Storyteller: body, illness and ethics.* Chicago, IL: University of Chicago Press; 1995.
13. Ibid.
14. Thomas, 2002, op cit.

15. Frank, op cit.
16. Parsons T. *The Social System*. New York, NY: Free Press; 1951.
17. Rogers CR. *A Way of Being*. Boston, MA: Houghton Mifflin; 1980.
18. John E. The Bridge. *The Captain and the Kid* [recording]. Mercury; 2006.
19. Bedingfield N. *Unwritten* [recording]. Arista; 2004.
20. Stevens C. Oh Very Young. *Buddha and the Chocolate Box* [recording]. Island; 1974.
21. Spence DP. *Narrative Truth and Historical Truth: Meaning and Interpretation in Psychoanalysis*. New York, NY: Norton; 1982.
22. Kermode F. *The Sense of an Ending: studies in the theory of fiction*. London: OUP; 1966.
23. Mattingly C. *Healing Dramas and Clinical Plots*. Cambridge: Cambridge University Press; 1998.
24. Ibid.
25. Yalom I. *Love's Executioner and Other Tales of Psychotherapy*. Harmondsworth: Penguin; 1989.
26. Pullman P. *The Amber Spyglass (His Dark Materials, Book III)*. London: Scholastic Books; 2000.

PART II

Introduction

Kleinman[1] points out that 'the study of illness has something fundamental to teach each of us about the human condition, with its universal suffering and death. Nothing so concentrates experience and clarifies the central conditions of living as serious illness' (p. xiii). Indeed, it could be argued that nothing confronts us with our human frailty quite like serious illness. From the unsettling beginnings of symptoms that lead us to consult a doctor, through tests, diagnosis, and treatment, there is major disruption to life. Pain, loss, disability and death raise fundamental questions about life, meaning, purpose and identity.

In the following chapters, I will examine particular aspects of the narratives in this book by looking across the stories through the lens of my personal responses and theoretical understandings; in this way, I aim to offer an interpretation of the narratives that complements the individual stories in Part One. In Chapter Six, I focus on the use of imagery by the storytellers; if identity formation is influenced by the dialectic and fluid relationship between culture and agency, then the stories we tell both shape and are shaped by the language we use. The stories in this study draw on a wide range of discourses, and are rich in imagery and analogy. Metaphor and simile are fundamental means by which we convey subjective experience and are both embodied as well as culturally informed.[2,3] An examination of the use of figurative language across all five stories will then illuminate the part this plays in the construction of experience and selfhood.

In Chapter Seven, I focus on the question, 'What dimensions of illness experience are highlighted by the stories?' Here I examine facets of the stories that reflect particular concerns and pertinent issues. Although each story is unique, everyone in this study shares the experience of illness that requires admission to hospital and also major surgery. Furthermore, each person's life has been permanently affected by his or her condition. The issues which these stories raise emerge from a commonality of experience, and therefore an examination of the issues presented by the storytellers may illuminate important human concerns. Sacks[4] writes of his post-encephalitic patients in *Awakenings*, 'It was necessary for them to find or make a life with individuality and dignity', and that while this was 'especially clear in these neurologically damaged patients', it also 'made clearer what is needed and sought by us all'[5] (p. 46).

REFERENCES

1. Kleinman A. *The Illness Narratives: suffering, healing and the human condition.* New York, NY: Basic Books; 1988.
2. Lodge D. *Consciousness and the Novel.* London: Secker & Warburg; 2002.
3. Lakoff G, Johnson M. *Metaphors We Live By.* London: University of Chicago Press; 1980.
4. Sacks O. *Awakenings.* London: Gerald Duckworth and Co; 1973.
5. Sacks O. Neurology and the soul. *New York Review of Books.* 1990; **37**(18): 44–50.

CHAPTER 6

Imagery

INTRODUCTION

The stories we tell regarding health and illness are rich in imagery and analogy, and draw on images from fields as diverse as war, machinery, technology, art, music, nature, landscape and travel.[1,2,3,4,5] My intention in this chapter is to explore the use of imagery and metaphor in the preceding stories. I start by looking briefly at imagery in literary and linguistic terms: at what metaphor does and how it works. I then examine the use of metaphor by the storytellers; this includes a creative and poetic exploration of the use of imagery in each person's stories, since I believe that the distillation of expression which poetry allows and the 'patterned language' of poetic form 'serves to concentrate and compress words into much more meaningful relationships with each other than in prose'[6] (p. 12) and thereby intensifies its representational power and analytic force. As Richardson[7] notes, 'settling words together in new configurations lets us see and *feel* the world in new dimensions. Poetry is thus a *practical* and *powerful* method for analyzing social worlds' (p. 933).

IMAGERY AND METAPHOR

'Imagery', according to Peck and Coyle[8] (p. 37), is, in literary use, a comprehensive term that refers to the figurative use of language; this use of language in a non-literal way includes simile and metaphor. While simile compares one thing with another using the words 'like' and 'as', metaphor describes one thing in terms of another and makes a direct link between two things which are seemingly unrelated.

The work of linguists Lakoff and Johnson[9] demonstrates how metaphor is 'pervasive in everyday life, not just in language but in thought and action' (p. 3). This grounding of our conceptual systems in metaphor affects our perceptions, thoughts, values and constructions of everyday reality. The 'metaphors we live by' are often culturally grounded; for example, linear metaphors such as the portrayal of life as a journey, which prevail in Western cultures, can structure our ways of conceptualising the world.[10] Indeed, such root metaphors are so embedded within language or culture that we scarcely realise they are metaphorical.[11] This contrasts with the more conscious use of metaphor as a literary device, where the Russian formalists regarded it as a means of challenging dominant conceptions of the social world. This 'defamiliarisation' or disruption of preconceptions serves to focus attention through incongruity and by making 'the familiar strange'[12] (p. 20).

In everyday life, metaphorical thinking enhances our ways of making sense of the world by making connections between dissimilar areas of life. In doing so, metaphor both challenges our conventional ways of thinking about the world and grounds our encounters with the unexpected in the already known. By enriching the meaning and force of ways of thinking and feeling, it allows the expression of the complexity of experience. We may use imagery drawn from our particular 'frame of reference' or worldview, which is informed by the wider culture as well as by personal history. As well as drawing on a stock of culturally available metaphors, we may also create metaphors from our 'felt-sense' (a term used by Gendlin[13] to denote a holistic sensation which he sees as residing in the body, but which also encompasses a sense of embodiment within a social world). Expression of the 'felt-sense' can often enable access to the 'edge of awareness'[14] or, in Polanyi's[15] term, the kind of 'tacit knowledge' that lies on that intuitive edge between what is consciously known and what is sensed as a kind of 'gut-feeling'. As Kirmayer[16] argues, our metaphors are grounded not only in social experience and interaction, but also, fundamentally, in bodily experience, where they occupy 'an intermediate ground between embodied experience and the overarching narrative structures of plots, myths and ideologies'[17] (p. 155). According to Jackson[18] (pp. 127–49), metaphor reveals and reflects 'the interdependency of mind and body, self and the world'.

METAPHOR IN ILLNESS

Imagery in health and illness frequently reflects concepts and values upheld within the wider culture; in the months following my own diagnosis, when surgery seemed out of the question and decline and death very likely, I remember being aware that the conventional 'wisdom' about serious illness was that one is supposed to fight. I was not at all sure how I might go about this supposed fight, with its implications of winning or losing. And I do not see my survival as victory. In a conversation with Pat about the battle imagery associated with illness, she beautifully debunked this myth of fighting; with characteristic humour, and her customary roar of laughter, she said: 'I didn't do anything—I just lay there!' Although such metaphorical thinking is pervasive in contemporary Western culture, we can choose to resist it: for example, John Diamond, in a weekly column in *The Times*, charted the course of his cancer and challenged the dominance of such battle imagery. In his book, *C: Because Cowards Get Cancer Too*, he wrote:[19]

I despise the set of warlike metaphors that so many apply to cancer. My antipathy to the language of battles and fights has nothing to do with pacifism and everything to do with a hatred for the sort of morality which says that only those who fight hard against their cancer survive it or deserve to survive it—the corollary being that those who lose the fight deserve to do so. (p. 10)

While such metaphors can be resisted and challenged, they can nevertheless have a powerful influence on our attitudes to illness and the embodied selves we construct and reconstruct. As Lakoff and Johnson[20] put it, 'Most fundamental values in a culture will be coherent with the metaphorical structure of most fundamental concepts' (p. 22). Socially sanctioned metaphorical concepts may or may not be useful to us in health and illness; we may use or encounter imagery which can evoke the power and complexity of illness experience, imagery which may liberate and enable the reconstruction of alternative identities, or alternatively, that which can constrain, dismiss or stigmatise. The stories we tell others about ourselves, as Bruner[21] observes, depend on 'what *we* think *they* think we ought to be like—or what selves in general ought to be like' (p. 66). The *metaphors* that underpin our modes of thinking both carry and perpetuate socially acceptable modes of being. Thus, for example, if we are expected to 'fight' illness, we can come to view ourselves as courageous or heroic in victory, or conversely as cowardly or weak in giving in.

As Susan Sontag[22] argues, in her essays *Illness as Metaphor* and *AIDS and its Metaphors*, we invest the metaphors we use in and about illness with meanings which can sentimentalise (for example, tuberculosis mythologised as romantic), or stigmatise. In her examination of the metaphors associated with TB and cancer, and subsequently AIDS, she powerfully demonstrates how the myths surrounding illness are embedded in and perpetuated by the metaphors we use, and how the attribution of qualities of malevolence and invasion contribute to the taboo of illness and can compound the fear, shame and isolation of illness; for example, the equation of cancer with a 'death sentence'. She writes: 'As long as a particular disease is treated as an invincible predator, not just a disease, most people with cancer will indeed be demoralized by learning what disease they have' (p. 7). In her preface to the first essay, she states: 'My point is that illness is *not* a metaphor' and 'the most truthful way of regarding illness … is one most purified of, most resistant to, metaphoric thinking' (p. 3).

While I agree that many of the metaphors that predominate in health and illness stories can stigmatise, I do not think it is possible to be 'purified' of them. As the importance of metaphor in human thought and language demonstrates, they are a fundamental and embodied way in which we represent experience. In her second essay, Sontag[23] acknowledges that 'one cannot think without metaphors,' while reminding us that there are 'some metaphors we might well abstain from or try to retire' (p. 91).

The reference I made in Chapter One to a seminar on neuroscience and education, in which the speaker compared those with brain injury to a television thrown from a window and smashed on the ground below, is a pertinent example of the use of imagery that is stigmatising and that separates the person from the body in a reductive and dismissive way. It is also a clear example of what imagery does, and how it works. Schafer[24] observes that metaphor implies and involves a storyline: 'What is called unpacking a metaphor is in certain respects much like laying out the kinds of story that are entailed by the metaphor' (p. 32). As a means of understanding why I found the analogy offensive, I tried 'unpacking' and examining its implications and the conceptual world it entailed.

Unpacking the 'smashed television' analogy

Mechanistic and objectifying	It is dismissive and disrespectful of the fact that this is a person. It objectifies the individual, takes away agency and represents the person as a passive object who is so damaged as to be not human
Irreparable	It implies the person is beyond repair, irretrievable, 'fit for the scrap heap'; a television would clearly never work again, and is therefore written off. So, it implies that those with brain injury are similarly written off.
Simplistic	A simplistic, deficit model of the brain that doesn't take into account the brain's 'plasticity' and capacity for adaptation. The image of plasticity refers to the brain's capacity to reform or develop new connections:[25,26,27,28,29,30,31] Sacks[32] reminds us of its 'capacity for the most striking adaptations, not least in the special (and often desperate) circumstances of neural or sensory mishap' (p. xiii). The brain is not 'programmed and static', but 'dynamic and active, a supremely efficient adaptive system geared for evolution and change, ceaselessly adapting to the needs of the organism—and its need, above all, to construct a coherent self and world, whatever defects or disorders of brain function befell it' (p. xiii). A simplistic mechanistic analogy disregards the role of agency, intentionality and consciousness in neuroplasticity.[33]
General	A gross general term that doesn't take into account the uniqueness and humanity of individual people nor the specificity and precise nature of brain injury.
Violent	A violent image reminiscent of tales of rock bands trashing hotel rooms.

While such unreflective and stigmatising use of metaphor can clearly constrain thinking and influence attitudes, it is perhaps also the case that in circumstances such as illness where we encounter the unknown, metaphor can allow us to express new and unfamiliar experiences in terms that render the unknown more familiar. If metaphor is often valued in literature for the way it 'makes the familiar strange', perhaps in the occurrence of illness it enables us to do the *reverse*: to make the strange familiar. When we encounter the *unknown*, *unfamiliar* and *inexplicable*, metaphor can help us to 'navigate uncharted territory'. Whether we create our own metaphors, or draw on root metaphors, the use of imagery enables us to relate the unknown or strange to that which is already known; by making the strange familiar, we can thus symbolise our encounters with the shock and uncertainty of serious illness. For example, Sibbett,[34] an art therapist, expresses through her art-work and writing her 'felt-sense' of meaningful and powerful images; she draws on culturally accessible and personally resonant imagery to represent her experience of cancer as 'a battle to the death' with a tiger. She viewed the 'struggle with cancer' as one that she could 'win or lose', and although 'the tiger bit didn't win, not that time anyway' (p. 232), she was aware it 'would accompany me for the rest of my life' (p. 229). In response to comments she encountered such as, 'Well we all know we're going to die sometime', she develops and extends the metaphor:

> Having been bitten by the tiger, perceived his fearsome size, felt its hot gaze, is qualitatively different from knowing there are tigers who will kill, yet not having personally encountered one (p. 233).

Kirmayer[35] points out that we can create metaphors which, though they 'lack the larger temporal structure of narrative', are 'no less persistent or powerful' (p. 155). They serve as 'fragments of poetic thought' and 'moments of evocative and potential meaning that serve as turning points, narrative opportunities, irreducible feelings and intuitions that drive the story onward' (p. 155). By drawing on the metaphors used by the storytellers in this study, I aim to explore and develop these 'narrative opportunities'.

THE DIVIDE: ILLNESS AS A WORLD APART

There are various metaphors associated with the onset and the diagnosis of serious illness: Sontag[36] writes of illness as 'the night-side of life', and states: 'Everyone who is born holds dual citizenship, in the kingdom of the well and in the kingdom of the sick' (p. 3), referring to both the separation between the sick and the well alongside the common humanity. Rita Charon[37] (p. 21) writes of this separation:

> The divide between the sick and the well is capricious, unpredictable, sometimes reversible but in the end irrevocable. It spares no-one. One hurtles with the speed of a fall down a mountain from one side of the divide to the other; one is turned by years-long, silent cell-by-cell malignant change into a person with cancer. The world is transformed after a diagnosis of serious illness, not only in the corporeal aspects of life—now with pain, now with pills, now with slippers, now with a

wheelchair—but in the deepest wells of meaning—now with limits, regrets, forced separations, final plans.

As a physician of immense experience and humanity, Charon has not forgotten that this 'divide' is arbitrary and, in a sense, illusory; we can experience either or indeed both sides of the chasm. She refers to a 'deep and nameless sadness'[38] (p. 17) that divides the sick and the well, and which is characterised by a 'jarring, jolting, inarticulate presence of dread' (p. 20). This sense of separation and isolation is expressed powerfully by the storytellers, and certainly has resonance for me; my own metaphor has been that of inhabiting another world: a 'world apart' that is separated from ordinary everyday life. In the following poem, which is drawn from all the stories, I have used the metaphor of 'belonging' in the world of illness and sought to capture a sense of what it means to inhabit that 'world apart':

Strange Belonging
I am a stranger in that strange place
I feel the loneliness of such strange belonging

I didn't want to belong to it
But I did belong to it

I don't want to belong to it
But I do belong to it

I don't want to belong in this world
But I have to

I don't want to get used to that place
But I have to

And yet there's familiarity in this strange belonging
This 'home' from home

I daren't get used to being at home
For I'll return to that place
I have to

If I live my life
How will I bear
the return to that place

To 'belong' in the world of the sick
Is to be separated from life
And I have to

'STRANGE BELONGING': UNPACKING THE EXTENDED METAPHOR

The title and the first line of this poem are taken from my associations of being admitted to hospital in 1993 and the diagnosis that followed my first brain scan. The phrase, 'strange belonging', is intended to evoke a sense of the estrangement I felt in being separated from my life, the people I love, and my home, as well as being in a place that was 'strange' to me in the sense of being unfamiliar. The use of 'belong' comes from Jan, who said of her re-admission to hospital: 'I didn't want to belong to it, but I did belong to it.' For Jan, 'it' represented a kind of security, a 'home from home' alongside a sense of separation from home and family over which she had no choice. The 'having to belong' refers to the loss of control that goes with diagnosis of serious illness and admission to hospital; it refers also to Pat's experience of being a patient and nurse on the same renal unit, to Jim's anxiety about being discharged from hospital, and to Yasmin's experience of spending so much time in hospital that she did not dare to adjust fully to her short spells at home.

PAT

Pat used the metaphor of 'everything turned on its axis' to denote her experience of the reversal of circumstance that sends her spinning into the world of the sick. She drew on positional metaphors of hierarchy; she felt 'demoted' and 'lower class', experiencing what Sacks[39] terms a 'reduced stationless status' (p. 122). It was also particularly difficult for her to undergo examinations from medical staff that she knew socially as well as professionally. As a patient, she experienced a loss of power and control; her sense of violation and of the rupture of personal boundaries are powerfully captured by her use of the metaphor 'a kind of rape', in which she was 'stripped bare' to 'her soul', 'naked' with 'nothing to hide behind'.

Pat uses 'alive' as a metaphor, declaring, 'I want to be "alive" in the sense of being "part of the world" and free from the "chains" of illness which "which pin and bind"'. Her metaphors are often profoundly embodied; she felt like a 'walrus' rather than 'a butterfly' who can 'flutter here and there'. Her transplanted kidney feels 'alien sometimes … like a separate entity'. I will discuss this further in Chapter Seven when I consider embodiment.

JAN

Jan talked of feeling 'alone' when she was readmitted to hospital in her teens. Part of the existential aloneness of her 'belonging' was that as a teenager she was on the cusp of independence, yet had no choice but to re-enter hospital; Jan potently captures this loss of choice and control through her use of 'Big Brother' as a metaphor. When she talks of the recurrence of pain in her hips, and of the need for hip replacement at some point in the future, she says, 'I don't quite want that Big Brother thing yet.'

The 'Big Brother' image, from Orwell's *1984*, represents surveillance, monitoring and loss of control. But it is ambiguous, for it also offers security and safety. 'Big Brother is watching you'[40] (p. 3), but this 'watching' has more than one meaning: we are being watched, but also watched *over*. As Jan says, 'If something's got to be done, somebody will be there to make the decisions for you and look after you.' Jan, though, is at a point in her life where she wants the independence and freedom to make her own choices, and being 'back in the system' would threaten that freedom: 'I don't want to get into a position where somebody else is making the decisions for me,' she says.

Jan uses the simile 'it felt like I had had my cotton wool ripped off from around me' to convey her loss of a layer of protection and her sense of vulnerability on leaving hospital and returning to school.

One of the most powerful and graphic images she uses conveys her 'felt-sense' when she observed an orthopaedic operation. She described this as 'a different kind of butchery', and returned to the image in a subsequent conversation:

A Different Kind of Butchery
I just had this sense of … oh god …
It just seemed …
Like a butchers shop really
And I remember thinking
Gosh …
I wonder what happened …
But not wanting to know…
It's just such an unreal experience
to see all these gowned up people
and this body …
and orthopaedic surgery
is very much … brutal
like a different kind of butchery

While her story sets the context—the overarching narrative—in which the 'butchery' metaphor is used, it is this graphic image that enables a glimpse of Jan's shock at witnessing a scene of orthopaedic surgery similar to her own, and which triggers her fleeting, 'Gosh, I wonder what happened'. Ricoeur[41] writes of the relationship 'between the figurative sense of the borrowed word and the proper meaning of the absent word' (p. 52). The power of Jan's use of 'a different kind of butchery' lies in the tension it evokes between the conventional or 'proper meaning' of the word 'butchery', referring to the slaughtering of animals for food, and its figurative use. In the generation of a metaphor that shocks, she conveys the impact of this experience in a way which recreates and communicates its power. It is a use of metaphor which exemplifies Ricoeur's distinction between the 'occasional causes of tropes', which involve a 'reduction of metaphor to a mere ornament' (p. 51), and 'the properly generative causes: imagination, spirit, passion,' which 'give colour, astonish, and surprise through new and unexpected combinations' (p. 73). At the same time, by expressing her sense of the unknown in terms of the known, Jan is making the strange familiar and grounding an encounter with the unexpected in a setting that is more recognisable and conventional.

JIM

Jim's choice of *Redemption Song* by Bob Marley[42] seemed to me to symbolise the ambiguous nature of his sense of freedom alongside his anxiety. As singer-songwriter Annie Lennox[43] has said of music, 'You identify with it, personalise it, it becomes a part of you'. Jim expressed his sense of vulnerability powerfully in his account of returning to work and drew on metaphors of size, and sequence: returning to work was 'massive' and 'everything seemed to be a first'.

There are many metaphors associated with our mortality. In the following poems, written entirely from Jim's words, I draw on the imagery he used to express the shock of diagnosis and of confrontation with his own mortality. The first poem, 'Dr Who?' uses a metaphor Jim drew from a popular BBC television programme.[44] He used this to describe his ascent into a mobile angiography unit; a world that evoked for him a sense of science fiction. The second stanza draws on the more mundane but equally evocative metaphor he used of a plumber, which conveys his 'felt-sense' of hearing the diagnosis of blocked arteries. Plumbing imagery is, as Hanne and Hawkin[45] note, frequently used by health professionals to 'explain to patients the nature of their cardiovascular or urinary tract problems' (p. 94).

Dr Who?
I was lifted up -
it was like going into the Tardis -
televisions everywhere
screens on the ceiling
A metal glare
a cold cold feeling.

Do you know that feeling?
When you get a plumber come
and he'll like tap your radiator
and go 'tut-tut … ooh'
Sharp intake of breath
Sucking of teeth
Eyes up in the air

This doctor
I shall never forget
I'm useless with names
But I'll always remember him

He had all the gear on
headphones
eye piece

All of a sudden
these screens just come alight,

My heart come up on the screen
I couldn't look

And he looked
And he said
 'You got arteries blocked
That artery's blocked
That one's blocked
And that one's no good
You need a bypass'

And there was me
thinking I was bullet proof,
and gonna live forever

In seeing his heart with its blocked arteries on the screen, Jim is brought face to face with his mortality, and the realisation he was not 'bulletproof'. In the following poem, Jim powerfully expresses the heightened sense of mortality that remains following life-threatening illness in the phrases 'the wall', 'the edge' and 'old bones':

Old Bones
When you've been to the edge
When you get to the point of no return
Which I got to
Make no bones about it

Once you've been to that wall
Everything becomes different
It's hard to explain to people
No one will ever understand
how it feels
when you've been to the wall

Closing your eyes
Going to sleep
not knowing if you're going to wake up

what can happen to you …
if you would ever wake up …
You can't explain that to anybody, can you?

You must recognise that feeling …
whereas someone who's never ever been there …

People just don't know
never understand
how it feels
once you've been to that wall
and how you live with that

There were times
when I thought
I'm not gonna make old bones.

Do you know what I mean?

As Bolen[46] notes, 'When life is lived at the edge—in the border realm between life and death—it is a *liminal* time and place'. (p. 15) This liminality and 'death salience', as Little and Sayers[47] describe it, are also experienced by Pat, Yasmin and by me. I will discuss these further in the next chapter.

Jim later talked about how his experience of illness has influenced his perspective on life, and he drew his metaphor 'tins of beans' from his work as a manager in one of the United Kingdom's supermarket chains (*see* Chapter Four). It is an example of metaphor as culturally contextualised, and also creative and enhancing in that it facilitated the construction of alternative identity.

There are other metaphors related to heart surgery such as the 'zipper club', which refers to the patient's scar. Although Jim referred to this metaphor, he didn't particularly draw on it. He used a range of images that were relatively militaristic, such as 'bulletproof' and 'marched'. The invasive nature of such surgery and his fear in the immediate aftermath that the incision in his chest could open up was powerfully captured in his use of the metaphor 'if you cough your chest must explode'.

YASMIN

The divide between the world of sickness and health was profound and unrelenting for Yasmin, as she struggled for the last 15 years of her life with the acute drama and the relentless day-in, day-out suffering of her severe inflammatory bowel disease. Her ileostomy and its many complications hugely intensified this division, incarcerating her cruelly in the land of the sick. The acute and enduring nature of her suffering powerfully prompted the questions 'why me?' and 'what have I done to deserve this?' The metaphor implicit in her questions is that of illness as punishment. She later made this explicit when she told me, 'I remember reading an article once which said that people suffer in their life because of the bad things they did in a previous life ... I don't believe it ... and I don't believe in God; I think if there was a god, how could he just stand by and see so much suffering.'

Nevertheless, the question remained for Yasmin:

Why?

Why do I bother?
What is the point?
I don't know why
I say to them,
Why is it happening to me?
And they say, "We don't know – 'cos you're different ... 'cos you're special."
I don't want to be different and special.
Why don't they know?
I just want them to get me better, you know?
Why don't they know?
Why is it so different for me?
What life have I actually got?
Why is it not my time?
Why am I being made to suffer so much?

Yasmin described how her 'sense of being part of the world was completely gone'. This was so profound that she felt barely 'alive'. This use of 'alive' takes on a metaphorical sense; although physically, biologically alive, she felt that she was just existing rather than engaging in the world.

Alive

It's like my life's over.
My sense of being part of the world
Gone
Being in hospital for so long
cocoons you

To emerge is hard
When you come out
Everything's just too much
The world's a scary place.

I spend so much time in hospital
I need to ...

If I come out and get used to the outside world
If I adjust too fully to living in the outside world
It would be harder to go back in

I've spent more time in hospital than out
My future is in and out of hospital
So I don't want to break that mould.

It's best if I'm in that frame of mind
But it's an awful way to be

I wasn't going to let illness control my life.
But it rules my life
It has to
The intravenous stuff
18 hours a day

This is no life
It's like *not* living my life

That sense of being 'part of the world' that Yasmin refers to is an extended metaphor—a use of 'alive' as metaphorical concept: 'That's it. My life's over', she tells her sister. 'I haven't lived my life' and 'illness rules my life' she tells me, for in the 'kingdom of the sick', she is both 'subject' and 'subject to' its claims and demands.[48] She uses the metaphor of hospital as a cocoon. This implies a stage of metamorphosis or transition; but for Yasmin, any emergence from the 'cocoon' of hospital is transitory, temporary and uncertain.

During a short period of respite, she drew on the metaphor of a bridge, and for a brief but fleeting time, felt that she had crossed over. 'The bridge', however, was precarious and fragile; it was always likely to give way, and send her crashing once again into the 'deep and nameless sadness'[49] (p. 17) of illness. The 'abyss at which patients routinely stand',[50] (p. 19) as Charon expresses it, held fear and hopelessness; it separated Yasmin from her family and friends, from the life she once had, from a life she could have had, and ultimately from her life at all.

As I was travelling home after meeting Yasmin for what was to be the last time, I listened to *Alive in the World*, a Jackson Browne[51] song that had particular resonance for me in the first years after my own illness. He sings of his desire to be a living, active and hopeful part of the world; his words and the poignant melody also seem to capture a glimpse of Yasmin's experience.

The language used in relation to health and illness is situated within a wider narrative context; metaphor is both embodied and also drawn from the discourses of literature, popular culture and the clinical setting. The plotlines, myths, and over-arching metanarratives of health and illness generate a range of metaphors that both inform and are informed by the experience of individuals. As Altschuler[52] notes, 'images and metaphors of our art, literature and everyday speech powerfully influence interactions between all players in the health system' to the extent that they 'construct the experience of illness for both professionals and families' and are 'linked with disparities in health care in Britain' (p. 7).

The metaphors used and encountered by the storytellers in this study are rich and diverse; they demonstrate how language use in the arena of illness experience draws heavily on existing metaphorical concepts but can also be creative and imaginative in ways which can express complexity, and enrich understanding. David Rennie[53] reminds us of the importance of listening for metaphors in the therapeutic setting, and also of allowing metaphoric resonance when we listen to others' stories. In experiential therapy, such as the person-centred approach, we might tentatively offer such resonance in the form of an image or metaphor as an expression of empathic understanding, congruence or acceptance.

Narrative approaches to therapy similarly draw attention to the use of imagery and metaphoric resonance, where they are particularly helpful as a means of enriching and thickening stories.[54] The use of 'reflecting teams' and outsider witnessing practices, developed by White[55,56,57,58] and subsequently by other practitioners (Payne,[59] Speedy[60,61,62]) draw on the work of Myerhoff,[63,64] in which 'definitional ceremonies' offer the opportunity for collaborative ways of enriching stories. The focus of these practices is not on evaluation, but on listening and retelling of stories by, for example, identifying 'what expressions and images from the story resonated with events or images within their own life'[65] (p. 106). As Speedy observes, such practices can 'seem quite countercultural', particularly in contemporary Western societies. However, such attention to the richness and nuances of language could contribute significantly to the quality of relating that Charon[66] advocates in the practice of 'narrative medicine'. Just as such practices are aimed at destabilising the power dynamics of the therapeutic setting in which the therapist is regarded as expert, so such attention to language could enhance the quality of the clinical encounter.

If we listen for metaphoric language, in ourselves and in others, we can become more aware of the meanings and power of particular analogies and challenge those that are unhelpful. Perhaps, we should not, as Sontag[67] first suggested, 'purify' illness talk of metaphorical thinking, but rather expand our range of available metaphors. The creative use of metaphor can facilitate the expression of multiple meanings and thus contribute to re-authoring stories which are closer to the actualities and complexity of experience and which can serve as 'narrative opportunities'[68] (p. 154), thereby restoring a sense of agency.

Imagery often indicates some of the common concerns and existential issues of illness experience. Some of these, such as embodiment, isolation and liminality, have been touched on in this chapter; in the following chapter, I will consider these in more detail.

REFERENCES

1. Broks P. *Into the Silent Land: travels in neuropsychology.* London: Atlantic Books; 2004.
2. Frank A. *At the Will of the Body.* Boston, MA: Houghton Mifflin; 1991.
3. Frank A. *The Wounded Storyteller: body, illness and ethics.* Chicago, IL: University of Chicago Press; 1995.
4. Sibbett C. An art therapist's experience of having cancer: living and dying with the tiger. In: Waller D, Sibbett C. *Art Therapy and Cancer Care.* Maidenhead: Oxford University Press; 2005. pp. 223–47.
5. Sontag S. *Illness as Metaphor.* New York, NY: Farrar, Straus and Giroux; 1989.
6. Peck J, Coyle M. *Literary Terms and Criticism.* London: Macmillan; 1984.
7. Richardson L. Writing: a method of inquiry. In: Denzin N, Lincoln YK, editors. *Handbook of Qualitative Research.* London: Sage; 2000.
8. Peck, Coyle, op cit.
9. Lakoff G, Johnson M. *Metaphors We Live By.* London: University of Chicago Press; 1980.
10. Ibid.
11. Goatly A. *The Language of Metaphors.* London: Routledge; 1997.
12. Bennett T. *Formalism and Marxism.* London: Methuen; 1979.
13. Gendlin E. *Focusing.* New York, NY: Everest House; 1978.
14. Gendlin E. The client's client: the edge of awareness. In: Levant R, Schlien J, editors. *Client-Centered Therapy and the Person-Centered Approach: new directions in theory, research and practice.* New York, NY: Praeger; 1984. pp. 76–110.
15. Polanyi M. *The Tacit Dimension.* Gloucester, MA: Peter Smith; 1983.
16. Kirmayer LJ. The body's insistence on meaning: metaphor as presentation and representation in illness experience. *Medical Anthropology Quarterly.* 1992; **6**(4): 323–46.
17. Kirmayer LJ. Broken narratives: clinical encounters and the poetics of illness experience. In: Mattingly C, Garro L. *The Cultural Construction of Illness and Healing.* Berkeley, CA: University of California Press; 2000. pp. 153–80.
18. Jackson M. Thinking through the body: an essay on understanding metaphor. *Social Analysis.* 1983; **14**: 127–49.
19. Diamond J. *C: because cowards get cancer too.* London: Vermilion; 1998.
20. Lakoff, Johnson, op cit.
21. Bruner J. *Making Stories: law, literature, life.* New York, NY: Farrar, Straus and Giroux; 2002.
22. Sontag S. *Illness as Metaphor and AIDS and Its Metaphors.* London: Penguin; 1991.
23. Ibid.
24. Schafer R. *Retelling a Life: narration and dialogue in psychoanalysis.* New York, NY: Basic Books; 1992.
25. Boller F. Rational basis of rehabilitation following cerebral lesions: a review of the concept of cerebral plasticity. *Funct Neur.* 2004 Apr-Jun; **19**(2): 65–72.
26. Edelman G. *Bright Air, Brilliant Fire: on the matter of the mind.* London: Penguin; 1992.
27. Luria AR. *Restoration of Function After Brain Injury.* New York, NY: Pergamon Press; 1963.
28. Sacks O. Neurology and the soul. *New York Review of Books*; 1990; **37**(18): 44–50.
29. Sacks O. *A Leg to Stand On.* Revised Edition. London: Picador; 1991.
30. Sacks O. *An Anthropologist on Mars.* London: Picador; 1995.
31. Schwartz JM, Begley S. *The Mind and the Brain: neuroplasticity and the power of mental force.* New York, NY: HarperCollins; 2002.

32. Sacks, 1991, op cit.
33. Schwartz, Begley, op cit.
34. Sibbett, op cit.
35. Kirmayer, 2000, op cit.
36. Sontag, 1991, op cit.
37. Charon R. *Narrative Medicine: honoring the stories of illness.* Oxford: Oxford University Press; 2006.
38. Ibid.
39. Sacks, 1991, op cit.
40. Orwell G. *1984.* London: Secker and Warburg; 1949.
41. Ricoeur P. *Time and Narrative.* Chicago, IL: University of Chicago Press; 1983.
42. Marley B. Redemption Song. *Uprising* [recording]. Island; 1980.
43. Lennox A. Desert Island Discs [recording]. 2008 May 11.
44. BBC Television. *Dr Who* [television programme]. 1963–present.
45. Hanne M, Hawkin SJ. Metaphors for illness in contemporary media. *Med Humanities.* 2007; **33**: 93–9.
46. Bolen JS. *Close to the Bone: life-threatening illness and the search for meaning.* 1998; New York, NY: Touchstone.
47. Little M, Sayers M. While there's life … hope and the experience of cancer. *Soc Sci Med.* 2004; **59**(6): 1329–37.
48. Sontag, 1991, op cit.
49. Charon, 2006, op cit.
50. Ibid.
51. Browne J. Alive in the World. *Looking East* [recording]. Elektra; 1996.
52. Altschuler J. *Working with Chronic Illness.* Basingstoke: Macmillan Press Ltd; 1997.
53. Rennie D. *Person-Centred Counselling.* London: Sage; 1998.
54. White M, Epston D. *Narrative Means to Therapeutic Ends.* New York, NY: Norton; 1990.
55. White M. *Re-authoring Lives: interviews and essays.* Adelaide: Dulwich Centre Publications; 1995.
56. White M. Reflecting team work as definitional ceremony re-visited. In: *Gecko: a journal of deconstruction and narrative ideas in therapeutic practice.* Adelaide: Dulwich Centre Publications; 1999.
57. White M. *Reflections on Narrative Practice: essays and interviews.* Adelaide: Dulwich Centre Publications; 2000.
58. White M. Re-Engaging With History: The absent but implicit. In: White M, editor, *Reflections on Narrative Practice: essays and interviews.* Adelaide: Dulwich Centre Publications; 2000.
59. Payne M. *Narrative Therapy: an introduction for counsellors.* London: Sage; 2002.
60. Speedy J. The storied helper: an introduction to narrative ideas in counselling and psychotherapy. *European Journal of Psychotherapy, Counselling and Health.* 2000; 3(3): 361–75.
61. Speedy J. Living a more peopled life: Definitional ceremony as inquiry into psychotherapy 'outcomes'. *The International Journal of Narrative Therapy and Community Work.* 2004; (3): 43–54.
62. Speedy J. *Narrative Inquiry and Psychotherapy.* Basingstoke: Palgrave Macmillan; 2008.

63. Myerhoff B. Life history among the elderly: performance, visibility and re-membering. In: Ruby J, editor. *A Crack in the Mirror: reflexive perspectives in anthropology.* Philadelphia, PA: University of Pennsylvania Press. 1982.

64. Myerhoff B. Life not death in Venice. In: Turner VM, Bruner EM, editors. *The Anthropology of Experience.* Chicago, IL: University of Chicago Press; 1986.

65. Speedy, 2008, op cit.

66. Charon, 2006, op cit.

67. Sontag, 1991, op cit.

68. Kirmayer, 2000, op cit.

CHAPTER 7

Issues

DIVERSITY AND SPECIFICITY ALONGSIDE UNIVERSALITY

Simone de Beauvoir[1] ponders questions of uniqueness and contingency and asks, 'Why am I myself?' She continues: 'What astonishes me ... is the fact of finding myself here, and at this moment, deep in this life and not in any other. What stroke of chance has brought this about? ... a thousand different futures have stemmed from every single moment of my past.' Indeed, what we all have in common is, paradoxically, our uniqueness: what makes us the same is our difference; we lead uniquely different lives subject to chance, contingency and particular combinations of biology, birth, life events, social and historical context, experience and choices. Each of the stories in this study reflects the particularity and diversity of individual experience and also gives insight into what it is to be ill in the United Kingdom in the late 20th and early 21st centuries. Perhaps the specificity of these stories also illuminates more universal concerns in relation to what it is to be human; as Kleinman[2] writes, 'Nothing so concentrates experience and clarifies the central conditions of living as serious illness' (p. xiii).

In this chapter, I will focus on particular themes that are highlighted by the preceding stories and examine the following issues which seem to me to encompass some of the chief concerns expressed by the storytellers: embodiment; depersonalisation; limbo.

EMBODIMENT

The relationship between self and body has been characterised in medicine and the social sciences by two relatively polarised positions. The naturalistic, biomedical model, which is based on Western mind/body dualism, focuses on the physical biological aspects of the body;[3] while the social, constructionist perspective regards the body as socially created and contingent on its social, cultural and historical context.[4] However, the notion of embodiment, which is rooted in the phenomenology of Merleau-Ponty,[5] refers to 'the lived body, our body being-in-the-world, as the site of meaning, experience and expression'[6] (p. 73). As a concept which emphasises the *intentionality* of being human as well as the lived experience of the person as material body, the notion of 'embodiment' provides a means of conceptualising personhood that challenges the Cartesian dualities of mind and body, and also takes into account biological and social factors.

Sparkes[7] asks himself the question, 'Do I *have* a body, or *am* I a body?' (p. 99). My own feeling is that in illness we perhaps come to know that we *are* bodies, though not just bodies: illness and health difficulties remind us that we are not separable but indivisible from our bodies. Embodiment is one of the conditions and challenges of life; our bodies are fundamental to who we are as persons. Much as we may at times want to separate from the sick body, our embodiment is a condition of our existence in the world, of life and of death. Illness underlines what Oakley[8] terms 'the universal, intensely perilous status of our bodies: biologically given, but subject at any moment to all sorts of cultural whims, misfortunes and outrageous attacks' (p. vi). When illness requires surgical intervention, as it has done for each of the storytellers, part of the shock and heightened awareness of our embodied state is that we require treatment which invades the boundaries of skin, bones, major organs and—through anaesthesia—transgresses consciousness itself.

Ultimately we are not machines to be fixed; we are people whose identities are personally embodied and socially embedded. Illness disrupts life and throws one's sense of self into disarray; we may wish to follow the cultural norm of 'getting back to normal', but with serious illness and long-term conditions, 'normal' is changed. For Yasmin, life was prematurely and profoundly changed, for Jan, it is inherently part of who she is—leaving her with the knowledge that her embodied condition will continue to interrupt her life. For Pat, whose transplant was eight years ago, there is a sense of borrowed time, and for Jim, there is another kind of normality in which healthy eating and exercise keep intimations of mortality at bay. For me, there is the legacy of left side pain and disability, and the MRI scan of my brain every two years.

All the storytellers began their narratives with their personal experience of being a 'body in the world': a body whose condition was in some way problematic and which required medical care and surgical intervention. Illness is primarily a reminder of our embodiment: a time when we cannot easily pretend that we are separate from our bodies. In good health, we can take our bodies for granted; they are seamlessly part of who we are. However, as the preceding stories show, when something goes wrong with our health, we become acutely conscious of our bodies. The body's apparent 'absence' in health becomes its abiding, inescapable and intrusive presence.[9] In everyday life, our bodies are often out of awareness, but illness, pain, dysfunction or accident can bring them sharply *into* awareness. As Murphy[10] expresses it, 'The body no longer can be taken for granted, implicit and axiomatic, for it has become a problem. It is no longer the subject of unconscious assumption, but the object of conscious thought' (p. 12).

The fragile status of the human body is universal: we are subject to our particular biological or genetic make-up, to the era, social conditions, class, time and place of our birth. Our bodies reflect and mediate cultural values and attitudes. When serious illness disrupts the workings of the body, causes impairment, and separates us from the life we knew, then our sense of continuity and order can feel threatened; we are reminded that we are, in Hamlet's phrase, subject to 'the slings and arrows of outrageous fortune', fragile, embodied and ultimately mortal. Illness intensifies the relationship between body and self as the body makes its presence felt through pain, discomfort, impairment and changes in appearance. In illness, the body is 'the front line' and the interface between ourselves and the world of medicine. It is, as Charon[11] notes, 'proxy for the self' (p. 86).

Pat's sense of embodiment was profoundly disrupted by her kidney failure. She was both the experiencing body and also, in Murphy's[12] words, the 'object of conscious thought' (p. 12). Her kidney failure meant that she had to restrict her diet, and dialysis made her reliant on a machine to do the work of her kidneys. As well as living the renal failure, she was evaluating and assessing her condition from the perspective of a practitioner. Her body was also the 'object of conscious thought' in the form of medical attention from her colleagues. What was private and intimate had become medical territory.[13,14]

The difficulty of altering her life and sense of self to accommodate physical losses and to reunify her body and selfhood was vast; not only was she feeling increasingly tired, breathless and nauseous, but the limitations that illness and treatment imposed on her life were impacting on so many dimensions of self. The additional complication of her heart problems further reinforced for Pat 'how fragile everything is'.

Wright and Kirby[15] note the effect of kidney failure on body-image, and so does the United Kingdom National Kidney Federation. The notion of 'body-image', according to Williams,[16] is a useful concept in that it 'links the biological, psychological and sociological levels of analysis' and 'implies the fundamental inseparability of mind and body' (p. 703). It is no surprise that the effects of transplant and immuno-suppressant drugs on Pat's body and on her self-image have been profound. Her body has undergone major physical changes; her dramatic weight loss and gain, together with the scars from her kidney transplant and heart operations, have combined with the changes associated with aging. Pat talked of her loss of confidence, and of social status, clearly describing and reflecting the gendered and age-related notions of the 'ideal' body.[17,18,19]

'It doesn't make you feel confident and also it's not acceptable to people's idea of health; people grade you and class you as to how healthy you are, same as when you're fat. People make judgements and you sink low in their estimation. Sometimes you catch yourself in a shop window and you think, oh God ...'

Failing health highlights the aging process for Pat: 'When you look at your body, it's like you've lost 20 years ... and the weight doesn't help either ... you do feel old.'

She distances herself from her body: 'I just feel it belongs to someone else, I don't think it's mine actually ... and when you see all these young girls with their smooth skins and beautiful decorated chests—I feel quite envious actually. I know I'm in my 40s, but still … you see old ladies and they've got beautiful skins … I'm quite disgusted with it. It's like a road grid; I've got so many scars … and people will stare. But I think, well no, I survived this … But it is a reminder of your mortality, a reminder of how fragile everything is.'

Weight gain and scars signify the disruption to Pat's body and to her life; they are important signifiers of what she has suffered but also indicate her survival. Implicit in the notion of embodiment is, of course, mortality, and Pat's scars signify her heightened awareness of this. 'Death salience', as Little and Sayers[20] term it, is 'the reflective awareness in a survivor that a mortal extreme experience could have led the subject down a fork in the road of serious illness to death and personal extinction' (p. 1334). A kidney transplant will only last for a limited time, so Pat cannot take her health for granted. In addition, she has heart disease. Therefore she has to be regularly monitored by both cardiology and renal specialists. At the present she is working in a community-based scheme to support those who live with long-term health problems. She prefers 'not to think too far ahead' and has found a way to live her life, but differently from the way she had expected or hoped.

A further complication of Pat's sense of embodiment was related to the transplant itself. She felt immense compassion for the donor and his family, as well as gratitude and humility, but also 'found it quite distressing at times to have a piece of somebody else in me … it felt abhorrent in a lot of ways; it does feel alien sometimes … like a separate entity'.

As Oakley[21] puts it, 'It's hard to dispose of the notion that, in incorporating bits of others' bodies into our own, we are also absorbing their identities'. (p. 118) Penny Amarena (personal communication, 2008) similarly notes this in relation to her research with transplant patients:

> Some participants felt they were influenced by the dead donor through the transplanted organ. There was an adaptive challenge to come to terms with thoughts and feelings about hosting an alien organ.

For Jan, the genetic nature of her condition meant that it was, as she said, 'fundamentally' and 'inherently me'. There was no 'before and after' the disruption of illness for Jan, since it was a dimension of her identity that was embodied at a microscopic, physiological level in her DNA codes[22] (p. 64). This particular genetic embodiment connecting her through the female line of her family carried for Jan a sense of responsibility. She could empathise with her mother, and knew that 'more than likely it will affect my children'.

At the same time she had a sense of 'my bones being mended by other people; of them not being natural', but 'almost man-made'. She described a sense of helplessness that accompanied this feeling of 'someone else having to make them better'. Her sense of embodiment therefore *incorporates* the 'man-made'. I use incorporate here deliberately in order to emphasise its sense derived from the Latin—*incorporare*—to 'put into or include in one body' (Oxford English Dictionary). And just as aging is fundamentally a process of embodiment, the pain in Jan's hips signals her embodied state and the prospect of further surgery as she gets older.

As with Pat, there were occasions and times in her life when Jan was conscious of her scars but also saw them as signifying 'what I'd been through'. Sibbett[23] similarly acknowledges her scars as 'special', and writes, 'I regard them as marks of survival' (p. 232). Jan's scars, while representing the disruption entailed by her embodiment, also signify the 'positive consequences' that have had a formative and valued influence in her life.

The scar held powerful associations for Jim of the invasive nature of heart surgery, directly conveying the sense that his body had been opened up, and reflecting his initial anxiety that it might 'explode'. Jim's sense of his own body as being fragile was a complete shock to him; he had regarded himself as 'fit and well', although his wife, he felt, 'had some inkling'. This reflects dominant notions of masculinity in which men have been portrayed in the media as 'neglectful of their health and childlike, requiring the care and attention of their partners'[24] (p. 28). Culturally available models of masculinity, which take for granted the view that men are inherently stronger than women, together with representations of 'men as oblivious to body-centred concerns such as health because of their preoccupation with work and their view of themselves as invulnerable to illness' (p. 29), can therefore have implications for how vigilant men are in monitoring their own health. Where the care of the male body is seen as the preserve of women, then men may be less attuned to signs of illness. In addition, responsibility for acting on such signs may also be delegated. It was the women in Jim's family whose persistence finally secured the angiogram he needed.

Jim was confronted with a sense of his own embodiment and its implicit mortality when he saw his blocked arteries on the screen, heard his diagnosis, and realised he wasn't 'bulletproof'. He powerfully expressed his realisation and heightened awareness of the fragile status of his body in his fears that if he went to sleep he 'might not wake up again'.

While according to Hession,[25] the National Service Framework for Cardiac Rehabilitation stipulates that there should be interventions to 'assist lifestyle changes, psychological adjustment, quality of life, social assessment and medical status' (p. 11), Thompson *et al.*,[26] found that cardiac rehabilitation services were incomplete, and, according to Bethell *et al.*,[27] 'less than a third of patients eligible for rehabilitation receive it'. Jim's experience of rehabilitation, however, was one in which his embodiment was recognised; he was offered both counselling as well as support from a multi-disciplinary team that offered information on diet, medication relaxation and strategies for dealing with stress. This holistic approach to rehabilitation, which took account of the many dimensions of embodiment, enabled Jim to reflect on his previous behaviour patterns and habitual ways of responding to stress, and offered him support in developing ways of 'exercising' control over his body. By following a regime of fitness and healthy eating, Jim has been able to actively engage in maintaining his own health.

Yasmin's suffering was so continuous and unremitting that illness 'ruled her life' for 15 years until her death; the long term, ongoing nature of her condition affected every dimension of her life. The everyday routines of toilet use and washing were fundamentally changed and served as a frequent and regular reminder of being differently embodied. In the case of ileostomy, as Kelly[28] observes, 'the symmetry of the body is changed. A new part which was not there previously is added, and the site of a major body function is altered and made visible in a way which when viewed from anything other than a medical perspective, is odd' (p. 397). As Etherington[29] notes, 'the silence surrounding these types of illnesses creates a sense of isolation and alienation for sufferers' (p. 11). The embarrassment and shame associated with incontinence meant that Yasmin no longer felt a sense of having an attractive, womanly, sexual body. The control and independent bodily status of taken-for-granted adulthood was further compromised by her need for intravenous nutrition and fluids.

In addition, there were occasions when she suffered extreme and intolerable physical pain, characterised by what Scarry[30] terms its ultimate 'unshareability' and 'resistance to language' (p. 4). Such pain is 'incontestably and unnegotiably present', and at its most extreme 'does not simply resist language but actively destroys it, bringing about an immediate reversion to a state anterior to language, to the sounds and cries another human being makes before language is learned' (p. 4). Try as we might, we cannot imagine ourselves into another person's physical pain and suffering, and there is a sense in which this underlines the isolation of human embodiment. Yasmin's survival through many occasions when she had been close to death implied both persistence in living alongside the acute fragility of her embodiment.

The heightened awareness of our bodies that comes with illness raises issues about 'qualia'—the specific nature of subjective experience—and accentuates the existential aloneness of our embodiment. For me, one of the aspects of being differently embodied is the sensory disturbance and neuropathic pain I experience on my left side. It is difficult to describe and to convey to others; in a sense it precedes language and in Levinas'[31] words, 'isolates itself in consciousness' (p. 176). There were times, as I was privileged to witness the stories told by Pat, Jan, Jim and Yasmin, when I was very conscious of the 'unshareability' of their suffering; times when words were not enough; times when I could not begin to imagine their suffering, let alone try to represent it; times when I could only be present with them in awe and respect. And I am aware of how difficult it must be for healthcare practitioners to witness suffering that they cannot ease.

Jaye[32] writes of general practice as being more open to the notion of the embodied experiencing person, and reports on the responses of GPs who explored the concept of embodiment as part of a medical anthropology course; she tells of the poignant and pertinent experience of one GP who, in a discussion of embodiment, described her medical training as 'ultimately disembodying in that it distanced her awareness from her own body so much so that she failed to recognise how disabling her asthma symptoms had become. It was also disabling in that she became alienated from patients as real and whole people' (p. 44). For this doctor:

> There wasn't time to think, there wasn't time to … be compassionate, you didn't have time to get to know people, you were running to physically keep up … I knew I had asthma but I didn't realise that's what was doing it and I couldn't understand why I felt exhausted all the time … It wasn't until things came to a head that I really went to see a respiratory physician who said, "you are bloody lucky you are not dead, what the hell did you think you were doing". It was that acute, so … you didn't really think about that. But I felt numb, I did feel distanced from my body, I felt withdrawn from sort of social contacts because it just took too much energy … I think you become less human.[33]

If the effect of medical training can be disembodying for the practitioner, then this may have an impact on his or her capacity to empathise with the patient, whose body may be seen more in terms of medical territory than as an embodied, experiencing person. Such 'disembodying' may then have the effect of 'depersonalisation'. As Campbell[34] notes, 'Allowing the medical narrative to include an awareness of the doctor's own bodily reactions might indeed transform medical practice. It could be a meeting place for the medical and lay narratives at those times in medical practice when what the patient or family needs is a humane understanding of a shared vulnerability' (p. 104).

It has been similarly valuable for me, as I have worked with the people contributing their stories to this study to remain aware of my own embodiment and tacit mortality. My scars and the deep crevices in my skull are a reminder to me of my own 'shared vulnerability'; they signify my survival and sense of mortality, but also connect me to others in shared humanity.

DEPERSONALISATION

Even if we accept the assertion that we *are* our bodies, this does not mean we are *only* our bodies. Although medical care at its worst can leave us feeling like physiological objects, at its best it can affirm a sense of shared humanity, even in the most desperate of circumstances. There is, however, as Sacks[35] puts it, a 'systematic de-personalisation which goes with becoming a patient …' (p. 28). Once we need medical care, we are defined as patients. On admission to hospital, one is tagged, asked to change into nightwear and slippers and shown to a bed; we become, as it were, inmates of the institution. There is a sense of passivity that inevitably accompanies diagnosis, medical care and hospital admission, and which contributes to the sense of being depersonalised. I think there are many reasons for this.

For myself, there was an initial feeling of sheer helplessness that came with the news of life-threatening illness. There is also the physical constriction of being confined to bed, to the ward and to hospital with its attendant rules, routines, procedures and examinations. There is a sense of being under scrutiny, and of being, in Jan's phrase, 'passive in the process'. I know on the many occasions when I have lain within the confines of an MRI scanner where my role is to be physically prostrate, motionless and passive, how strongly I have wanted to be standing alongside the radiologists as they scrutinise images of my brain.

Each of the storytellers has underlined a need to be related to as a person and has deeply appreciated the occasions and the relationships within the medical setting when they felt recognised as people, with—to quote Murakami[36]—'a face, a life, a family, hopes and fears, contradictions and dilemmas' (p. 6).

The feeling of being 'defined' by illness and its accompanying depersonalisation was experienced by Pat as a 'demotion' from her status as nurse, where 'you're not a person … you're a patient … you're in that bed'.

Jan had felt at times defined by her bodily status, and regarded as 'the hip problem, not Jan'. This was particularly evident for her on occasions when she felt unacknowledged as a person with feelings and possibilities in her life.

The loss of personal privacy and focus on the body as the 'object' of medical attention was not only depersonalising, but was experienced by Pat, as a 'kind of rape', and by Jan as violation: in the following description of the ward round, Jan clearly shows how certain rituals that are embedded in the culture of hospital care can be experienced not only as objectifying but also violating:

> I'll never forget the time when I was 15 or 16 and lying in my knickers on the bed
> waiting for the ward round and having 10 medical students open the curtains. I
> remember that being very intrusive, and I was absolutely mortified; it felt like my
> privacy, my body, me, had been violated in some way …

Jan found 'that sense that people can just do that to you … quite a depersonalising process'. Such insensitivity and lack of respect for personal privacy left her feeling both 'violated' and 'powerless'. As she stated, 'I don't really think that sort of humiliation should be the norm'.

When I asked Pat what she wanted to come out of this research, she said she wanted practitioners 'to remember this is a person not an illness', and that 'the illness does not represent all that a person is'. She felt that this recognition would contribute greatly to being 'treated as an equal' by practitioners.

The severity of Yasmin's illness was such that it dominated her life and left her feeling defined as a patient, deprived of personhood, and reduced to a bodily status marked by difference, not only to those who were well, but to others with less severe IBD. While she recognized the sense of helplessness experienced by some practitioners in the face of her suffering, she had nowhere to direct her sense of injustice about this illness, and at times it seemed to her as if she had been abandoned. With no grounds or reason for hope, she felt the frustration of her doctors and the difficulties they faced in trying to relieve her immense suffering. But hope had long since deserted her, and in her words 'I'm a person too' I heard the echo of her voice in the wilderness of her inescapable embodiment.

In a paper exploring the place of narrative in serious illness and 'bodily conditions for which there is no biomedical cure'[37] (p. 73), Mattingly argues that narrative may be enacted rather than simply told, and that even when cure is not possible, 'performed narratives can have healing potential', and stresses that 'healing is not, it must be restated, synonymous with curing' (74). Yasmin conveyed a sense of this when she talked about her relationship with her counsellor:

> When they first offered me counselling I thought what do I want with a counsellor? And I resisted it for a couple of years. And then I thought, just to shut them up, I'll go once; and just being able to talk to her about how I feel, just being able to say it out loud. It's almost, although I can't fix it, being able to talk about it is almost as good. From the very first time I saw her I just felt I could tell her anything and everything and I did. I'm really surprised actually. I was saying things to Claire that I didn't even know myself I was feeling.
>
> And she has never ever told me you shouldn't feel that. She's never said you're wrong. Even when I said to her I feel suicidal she didn't say, oh Yasmin you shouldn't feel that, you should feel lucky for what you've got. She never ever said that's wrong to feel that ... looking back there were times when if it wasn't for her I don't know how I would have got through a situation. Just the fact that I know I can say anything to her, and it stays with Claire. And other times I've gone in and I've said well I'm in this situation but if I say something I'm not sure ... And she's gone and spoken to the doctor on my behalf. She really genuinely cares. And just having that, just knowing that there's someone there who really genuinely cares makes a difference. I don't know what I'd do without her really.

When illness is as protracted and unrelenting as Yasmin's, and when there is no possibility of resuming the life as once lived, then threats and challenges to personhood are acute. This underlines the fundamental importance of practitioners recognising the person in the midst of illness and suffering, and taking into account not just the physicality of the body but the life it represents. As a nurse who read Yasmin's story commented, 'This should be read by the nurses on the ward—they tend to forget that this is a person with a life.'

When practitioners do relate to us as persons, it is often the 'small moments' that can make a difference. Mattingly[38] writes, 'I have grown to respect and even to wonder at the power of small moments' (p. 76). Examples of such 'small moments' include Pat's surgeon, who was 'very hands-on' and rang to talk to her when he was unable to do the transplant until the following day; the cleaner Jan remembered who made the children laugh; Jim's nurse who gave him small pieces of bread when he felt nauseous; Yasmin's doctor who stood by her even when her suffering was most difficult to relieve. Particular moments I remember were the quiet empathy of my GP who listened to my despair when death seemed very probable. Another moment was when my surgeon detailed the high risks involved in my operation. When I asked, 'And death?' he silently inclined his head; then, as he stood up to leave, he offered me a glimpse of hope with his words, 'I will move heaven and earth to give you the best chance of coming through this'.

As Mattingly notes, such 'healing encounters are often well hidden from view' (p. 77); nevertheless, when serious illness disrupts life, those encounters can play an important part in compassionate clinical care and point to the fundamental importance of recognising the person who is more than this body, this illness or these symptoms, as well as the significance of the relationship between the sick person and medical practitioner.

LIMBO

Becker[39] (pp. 119–135) writes of the sense of limbo following disruption such as illness, and draws on Turner's concept of liminality[40] (1969), which signifies a threshold or social space between ways of being. Sibbett[41] similarly draws on Turner's conceptualisation of liminality to explore her own 'embodied and sensory experience of cancer' (p. 50).

There are many ways in which illness casts us into a state of limbo. As patients, we can spend a lot of liminal time and space in waiting rooms. There is often a period of waiting for appointments, tests, results, diagnosis or treatment, in which we can feel suspended in a state of uncertainty. It is widely recognised that for the person who is ill and for their friends or family, 'waiting is the worst thing'. As I write this, I am currently four weeks into the wait for the results of my last MRI scan. The passivity and powerlessness that accompanies this waiting is something I find particularly difficult. Indeed, Turner[42] regards passivity, 'submissiveness and silence' (p. 103) as characteristics of liminality.

With a long-term or possibly recurrent condition, there is a continual sense of uncertainty, where at some level we monitor our symptoms for possible change; a limbo that was for Sibbett[43] an experience of 'waver(ing) in liminality, living and dying with the tiger' (p. 223).

There is a sense of limbo when we are well enough to leave hospital, but too ill or too weak to participate in the outside world, or resume any form of 'normality'. Illness disrupts, constrains and confines our ways of 'being in the world'; we not only lose confidence in our physical bodies, but in our sense of ourselves as social beings. Sickness involves physical and emotional vulnerability, and brings a return to childlike dependency. The grown-up, and big, wide worlds of work, of socialising with friends, of holidays and walks, of gardening, of watching or playing sport, can seem out of reach and unattainable. Pat had talked of 'an erosion (of confidence) that happens from the moment you are diagnosed'. Illness can shrink our world; there is physical confinement to that bed, or that chair, those four walls, and that existence; the early steps out of that contracted world are necessarily tentative and cautious. The essence of convalescence, according to Sacks'[44] experience following his leg injury, was not just physical but lay 'in the whole general realm of coming to life, emerging from self-absorption, sickness, patienthood, and confinement, to the spaciousness of health, of full being, of the real world' (p. 121).

Jim experienced anxiety and a sense of acute vulnerability in this emergence from patienthood. Each of the 'massive firsts' he encountered were transitional stages, or rites of passage;[45] his move from HDU back to the ward, his first tentative and unsteady steps, his anxiety when leaving hospital and walking through 'those big green doors' on his return to work, all represented thresholds to be crossed, and transitions from one stage to another.

For many ill people, the state of limbo is one of estrangement from both the person they had been, and the life they had lived; it is, in Turner's[46] words, 'not any place they were in before nor yet any place they would be in' (p. 25). The last 15 years of Yasmin's life were characterised by an acute sense of limbo in which she was 'neither here nor there', but 'betwixt and between'[47] (p. 95). Separated from the life she had previously lived, and constantly in more often than out of hospital, she felt 'this is no life'. In my experience, serious illness can feel like a suspension from 'real life'; it is a twilight world on the margins of healthy and robust everyday life; a liminal space between a world of possibilities and potentialities, and one of doubt, uncertainty and suffering. For Yasmin, it was a twilight world from which she only ever fleetingly emerged; her brief glimpses of everyday life were tinged with an awareness that 'my future is in and out of hospital' and that the freedom to live her life was too much for which to hope. As Kleinman[48] observes, such limbo is 'a realm of menacing uncertainty' and isolation. He continues, 'Social movement for the chronically ill is back and forth through rituals of separation, transition, and reincorporation, as exacerbation leads to remission and then circles back to worsening, and so on' (p. 181). Such perpetual transition and uncertainty represented a permanent state of limbo in which Yasmin was constantly confronted by the existential challenges of life—freedom, search for meaning, isolation and inevitable death, Yalom's four 'givens of existence'.[49,50] Her suffering was without meaning or respite; it was, in Levinas'[51] words, 'intrinsically meaningless and condemned to itself without exit' (p. 158). Bolen[52] writes of life-threatening illness, 'When life is lived at the edge—in the border realm between life and death—it is a liminal time and place'. (p. 15) Part of the tragedy of Yasmin's death was that she spent the last years of her life inhabiting this liminal space.

REFERENCES

1. de Beauvoir S. *All Said and Done.* London: Andre Deutsch; 1974.
2. Kleinman A. *The Illness Narratives: suffering, healing and the human condition.* New York, NY: Basic Books; 1988.

3. Salmon P. *Psychology of Medicine and Surgery: a guide for psychologists, counsellors, nurses and doctors.* Chichester, NY: Wiley; 2000.
4. Nettleton S. *The Sociology of Health and Illness.* London: Polity Press; 1995.
5. Merleau-Ponty M. *The Phenomenology of Perception.* London: Routledge; 1962.
6. Gabe J, Bury M, Elston MA. *Key Concepts in Medical Sociology.* London: Sage; 2004.
7. Sparkes A. *Telling Tales in Sport and Injury.* Champaign: Human Kinetics; 2002b.
8. Oakley A. *Fracture: Adventures of a Broken Body.* Bristol: The Policy Press; 2007.
9. Leder D. *The Absent Body.* Chicago, IL: University of Chicago Press; 1990.
10. Murphy R. *The Body Silent.* London: WW Norton; 1990.
11. Charon R. *Narrative Medicine: honoring the stories of illness.* Oxford: Oxford University Press; 2006a.
12. Murphy, op cit.
13. Deleuze G, Guattari F. *A Thousand Plateaus.* London: Athlone Press; 1987.
14. Frank A. *The Renewal of Generosity.* Chicago, IL: University of Chicago Press; 2004.
15. Wright SJ, Kirby A. Deconstructing conceptualisations of adjustment to chronic illness. *J Health Psychol.* 1999; **4**(2): 259–72.
16. Williams SJ. Medical sociology, chronic illness and the body: a rejoinder to Michael Kelly and David Field. *Sociol Health Illn.* 1996; **18**(5).
17. Oakley, op cit.
18. Lupton D. *Medicine as Culture.* 2nd ed. London: Sage; 2003.
19. Becker G. *Disrupted Lives: how people create meaning in a chaotic world.* Berkeley and Los Angeles, CA: University of California Press; 1999.
20. Little M, Sayers M. While there's life … hope and the experience of cancer. *Soc Sci Med.* 2004; **59**(6): 1329–37.
21. Oakley, op cit.
22. Williams, op cit.
23. Sibbett C. An art therapist's experience of having cancer: living and dying with the tiger. In: Waller D, Sibbett C. *Art Therapy and Cancer Care.* Maidenhead: Oxford University Press; 2005. pp. 223–47.
24. Williams, op cit.
25. Hession J. At the Heart of Change: the impact of cardiac surgery on men's lives. Unpublished MSc [thesis]. University of Bristol; 2003.
26. Thomson DR, Bowman GS, Kitson AL, *et al.* Cardiac rehabilitation services in England and Wales: a national survey. *Int J Cardiol.* 1997; **59**(3): 299–304.
27. Bethell H, Turner J, Evans J, *et al.* Cardiac rehabilitation in the United Kingdom. *J Cardiopulm Rehabil.* 2001; **21**: 11–115.
28. Kelly M. Self, identity and radical surgery. *Sociol Health Illn.* 1992; **14**(3): 390–415.
29. Etherington K. Foreword. In: Thomas G. *Counselling and Reflexive Research in Healthcare: working therapeutically with clients with inflammatory bowel disease.* London: Jessica Kingsley; 2009.
30. Scarry E. *The Body in Pain: the making and unmaking of the world.* New York, NY: Oxford University Press; 1985.
31. Levinas, E. Useless suffering. In: Bernasconi R, Wood D, editors. *The Provocation of Levinas: rethinking the other.* London: Routledge; 1988. p. 158.
32. Jaye C. Talking around embodiment: the views of GPs following participation in medical anthropology courses. *Med Humanities.* 2004; **30**: 41–8.
33. Ibid.

34. Campbell AV, Willis M. They stole my baby's soul: narratives of embodiment and loss. *Med Humanities.* 2005; **31**: 101–4.

35. Sacks O. *A Leg to Stand On.* Revised Ed. London: Picador; 1991.

36. Murakami H. *Underground.* London: Vintage; 2003.

37. Mattingly C. Performance narratives in the clinical world. In: Hurwitz B, Greenhalgh T, Skultans V, editors. *Narrative Research in Health and Illness.* Oxford: Blackwell Publishing; 2004.

38. Ibid.

39. Becker, op cit.

40. Turner V. *The Ritual Process: structure and anti-structure.* Ithaca, NY: Cornell University Press; 1969.

41. Sibbett, op cit.

42. Turner V. *The Ritual Process: structure and anti-structure.* New York: Aldine de Gruyter; 1995.

43. Sibbett, op cit.

44. Sacks, op cit.

45. Van Gennep A. *The Rites of Passage.* London: Routledge and Kegan Paul; 1960.

46. Turner V. *The Anthropology of Performance.* New York, NY: Performing Arts Journal Publications; 1988.

47. Turner, 1995, op cit.

48. Kleinman, op cit.

49. Yalom I. *Love's Executioner and Other Tales of Psychotherapy.* Harmondsworth: Penguin; 1989.

50. Yalom I. *Existential Psychotherapy.* New York, NY: Basic Books; 1980.

51. Levinas, E. Useless suffering. Cohen RA, translator. In: Bernasconi R, Wood D, editors. *The Provocation of Levinas: rethinking the other.* London: Routledge; 1988. p. 158.

52. Bolen JS. *Close to the Bone: life-threatening illness and the search for meaning.* New York, NY: Touchstone; 1998.

PART III

Introduction

In Parts One and Two of this book, I represented five stories of illness. In a sense, the representations in Chapters One to Seven embody the methodological approach I have taken to this narrative inquiry. In Chapters Eight to Ten, I unpack the methodology I used. Readers who are particularly interested in the theory and methodology will find a more detailed account online, where I offer an examination of the philosophical ideas, assumptions, and values that underpin narrative, and also describe the development of my approach to narrative inquiry. Supplementary material relating to chapters Eight to Ten is available at: www.radcliffepublishing. com/devnarrativehcres/

The stories on which this research is based were informed by particular theoretical, philosophical and methodological values and concerns; in Part Three, I address these considerations and focus on the wider theoretical issues that underpin the research and inform the representations in Parts One and Two.

In Chapter Eight, I offer a rationale and justification for narrative as a methodology; here I show how assumptions about knowledge, and how we regard what it is to be human, influence and inform researcher positioning.

In Chapter Nine, I focus on how I carried out the research: my relationships with the people who took part, procedural and practical issues, questions of ethics and accountability, and how we might evaluate this kind of approach.

In Chapter Ten, I address questions of representation, writing and analysis, showing how the underlying rationale and method are reflected in the stories in Parts One and Two.

In Chapter Eleven, I consider some of the implications this research may hold for healthcare practice.

In the final chapter, I reflect on what I have learnt as I have made the transition from counsellor to researcher.

In my closing reflections, I return to my personal, autoethnographic voice.

CHAPTER 8

Narrative ideas: a rationale

INTRODUCTION

In this chapter, I examine what it is about narrative that is important for us as human beings and address questions of justification: questions of why I used a narrative approach to research illness experience and its impact on identity. I go on to outline some of the key ideas which inform narrative inquiry.

Narrative approaches to research have been developed across many disciplines within the health and social sciences and have gained increasing credibility as methods that capture personal and human dimensions of experience; they also incorporate contemporary critical thinking in a way that takes account of the relationship between individual experience and cultural context.

Research in health and illness is at the interface of science and life; since I set out to contribute research which embodies personal meanings and intentions, which expresses the uniqueness of each person and the particularities of experience as well as its social dimensions, then it was crucial to develop a methodology that would enable the telling of individual stories of illness and its impact on identity. Furthermore, this would require a means of representation that would both honour the particularities of lived experience and also encompass thematic and conceptual dimensions of illness. My intention was to explore the subjective experience of illness in all its immediacy, particularity and partiality; I was interested in what it was like to live 'this life' with 'this illness', and how living 'these experiences', with their shifts and changes, disruptions and transformations, influenced each person's sense of who s/he is and who s/he may become over time. Because my interest was in subjective experience, meaning-making, and sense of self, as well as in the issues raised by the personal stories, this required a methodology based on the principles and values of narrative approaches to human experience as lived and told stories, as well as on conceptual approaches to knowledge.

NARRATIVE

It has been claimed across many disciplines that it is fundamentally through narrative means that we make sense of our lives: that stories are not peripheral, but central and fundamental to our way of making meaning. Indeed, some recent work[1,2] on consciousness suggests that we have a predisposition towards story-telling which is 'hard-wired' into our brains. While I am a little wary of such fundamentalist claims, I agree with Polkinghorne[3] in his emphasis on the role of narrative in meaning-making, temporality and agency, which he describes as follows: 'Narrative … provides a framework for understanding the past events of one's life and for planning future actions. It is the primary scheme by means of which human existence is rendered meaningful' (p. 11).

Psychologist Jerome Bruner has argued that we have two different ways of knowing the world: paradigmatic, or logico-scientific knowing, which involves abstract, conceptual thinking; and narrative knowing, which is based on the way in which we organise and communicate experience through stories. According to Bruner,[4,5,6] our capacity to narrate develops almost as soon as we acquire language; from an early age, we are intuitively aware of how to tell stories. While paradigmatic approaches to knowledge, which emphasise conceptual and abstract models of reality, have long had greater status than stories in academic discourse, both are necessary means of making sense of human experience; our understanding of the world involves interplay between these two modes of thinking.

More recently, Bruner[7] has written of feeling 'uneasy with the answers I've come up with' in terms of 'comparing the narrative mode of thought with the logico-paradigmatic' (p. 115). He reminds us, 'Even etymology warns that "to narrate" derives from both "telling" (*narrare*) and "knowing in some particular way" (*gnarus*)—the two tangled beyond sorting' (p. 27). Etymologically, then, 'narrative' combines recounting of events with a particular kind of knowledge or understanding of them. This, I think, indicates the characteristics of narrative that go beyond sequencing of events and towards meaning-making.

The literary origins of the current interest in narrative go back to Aristotle, who suggested that stories have three key elements: events and actions unfolding over time; plot (which is to do with meaning and causality); and trouble, or 'peripeteia', in which 'a sudden reversal of circumstances swiftly turns a routine sequence of events into a story'[8] (p. 5). Stories focus on the particularities of experience and locate it in time and place. Bruner[9] stresses the inherent sequential nature of narrative and its focus on departure from the expected: 'the forging of links between the exceptional and the ordinary' (p. 47). The onset of serious illness is just such a departure from the ordinary, and the questions it raises; as Pat puts it, 'One day you're just pootling along and then the next …' The stories in this book are about such challenges, and the interpretations and meanings made from the intrusion of the exceptional into the expected. For 'the circumstance of story', as Bruner writes, is that 'it involves both a cultural convention and a deviation from it that is explicable in terms of an individual intentional state' (p. 51).

Bruner[10] uses a landscape metaphor to describe how stories operate: the 'landscape of action' is concerned with events over time and in context, and the 'landscape of consciousness' is concerned with meanings and values. These landscapes, according to Bruner,[11] are intertwined such that 'a narrative models not only a world but the minds seeking to give it meaning' (p. 27). For example, in my own illness story in Chapter One, I was not only putting my experience into words, but, through the filter of language, I was representing a *perspective* that signified the self I was telling. I was also enabling the evolution of that self through the telling process. As a counsellor, my experience of listening to and engaging with stories was often one of witnessing and participating in their transformative and constitutive power. There is literature from many therapeutic approaches to substantiate the ways in which narrating is not only healing, but constitutive of self.[12,13,14,15,16]

In *Trauma, the Body and Transformation*, a collection of moving and powerful stories, Etherington[17] clearly demonstrates how the telling of stories enables the evolution and creation of new ways of being. Arthur Frank's[18] work is additionally a powerful testament to the capacity of narrative as a way of reclaiming, transforming, and refashioning the self in illness.

NARRATIVE AS INTERSUBJECTIVE

As *relational* beings, we don't just *tell* stories, we tell them *to* someone (even if it is only ourselves). Narrating stories plays a vital role in personal and social relations and in our capacity for a compassionate and socially responsive life. Stories call forth stories in response. When we hear stories that are not usually or easily told—stories that step outside the well-rehearsed storylines of habitual discourse—we find resonance and 'gain permission' to respond with our own stories. When my story was published, people responded by telling me their illness stories, or those of family members. I heard, and also read, medical practitioners' stories. As a result of the dialogues my story opened up, there were changes made to medical practice. The people who have contributed their stories to this study have done so as an act of generosity—to me and also to others whom their stories might help. Telling stories is an ethical act, a moral standpoint, and creates space for others to enter into relation as fellow sick person, as medical practitioner, and above all, as fellow human being.

To back up that last point from my research, and to address the question 'why narrative?' a nurse who read one of my contributors' stories commented, 'This should be read by the nurses on the ward—they tend to forget that this is a person with a life.' When I asked my contributors what message they particularly wanted to get across, everyone indicated the importance of being recognised as a person. Charon[19] stresses the importance of medicine's attention to the uniqueness or 'singularity' of the person (p. 47) and shows how the relational and respectful approaches fostered by 'narrative medicine' enable the recognition that this is a person with, in Haruki Murakami's[20] words, 'a face, a life, a family, hopes and fears, contradictions and dilemmas' (p. 6). The recognition by the nurse above that 'this is a person with a life' demonstrates narrative's intersubjective capacity and transformative power. The relational dimension of narrative encompasses both our singularity and our shared humanity. I would add that if we learn to *tend* our own stories, and to acknowledge our own vulnerabilities, then we are more likely to *attend to* and to bear witness to the stories of others. This reflexive narrative process therefore not only leads inwards but outwards to others.

It is in the intersubjective space between self and other, which Martin Buber terms the 'I-Thou'[21] of relationship, that stories are heard and told. When we 'listen with' stories and allow resonance and connection as well as awareness of difference and uniqueness, then we may enable the telling of stories that may not otherwise be told: alternative stories, parallel stories, new stories, surprising stories, paradoxical stories. If narrative is constitutive of self, it is in relation to others that identity emerges. As Bronwyn Davies[22] writes, 'Listening to others tell their stories helps fill in the gaps and silences of knowing oneself as an embodied being' (p. 14). She writes of the collective storytelling process as one of 'tuning into oneself as an embodied being, to the emotion of it, and to the politically contested nature of it'[23] (p. 51): stories implicitly convey sociocultural relations. Storytelling is thus an interpersonal and social 'transaction' where we draw on the social and political discourses in which we are embedded as well as personally embodied.

NARRATIVE AND THERAPY

In his comprehensive review of the development of narrative ideas and their role in psychotherapy, McLeod[24] clearly shows how the different theoretical approaches to therapy have used the concept of narrative in distinct ways. The three principal approaches that draw on narrative have been the psychodynamic, the cognitive/constructivist and the social constructionist. The first two, in McLeod's view, 'are inserting the concept of narrative into existing theoretical frameworks' (p. x), and regard stories as a 'source of clinical data' and means of diagnosis. The latter 'places a sense of the person as a story-making and story-consuming being right at the centre of its conceptual framework'. McLeod views narrative approaches to therapy as principally associated with social constructionist thinking and terms them 'postpsychological' in that they challenge the concept of the unitary, bounded self with a view of the person as more fragmented and as socially constructed. This view emphasises the social, historical and cultural construction of reality through language and raises questions about the dominant stories through which we construct our social world; it also implies that we can choose to challenge or re-author them. Narrative therapy, he writes, 'forms part of a broad movement that has recognised the extent to which psychological models and concepts have contributed not only to the diffusion of what Kenneth Gergen has called a "language of deficit"[25] (p. 353) but also to the erosion of collective and communal forms of life and being in relationship'.[26]

The post-structural approach to narrative therapy of White and Epston[27,28,29,30,31] draws particularly on the theories of Michel Foucault[32] on power and knowledge and the way that these shape lives. The way in which 'constructed ideas are accorded a truth status'[33] (p. 19) is 'normalising' in that it leads people to define who they are and thereby constrain their lives according to social norms. For example, in Chapter Two, Jan reflects on the relationship between the normalising and dominant narrative in British society of 'get over it' and 'get back to normal' and her experience of orthopaedic surgery during childhood and adolescence.

In line with this emphasis on the interplay between personal agency and socio-cultural context, narrative approaches thus challenge the status and authority of the metanarratives[34] of the modern scientific era and value 'local', experiential knowledge and individual stories *alongside* the 'authoritative truth'[35] of these dominant narratives. The term 'local knowledge' is from the work of anthropologist Clifford Geertz[36] and refers to knowledge drawn from immediate concrete experience, which values personal meaning over 'expert knowledge', the two often fashioning and shaping each other in a dialectical fashion. The metaphors of structure and depth, which were drawn from hydraulics and characterised the psychology of Freud and others, have been similarly challenged, and alternative metaphors such as thickness or richness have been used. Geertz draws on the thick/thin metaphor, originated by philosopher Gilbert Ryle,[37] which refers to the intentions and understandings of actors as opposed to the unexamined preconceptions of observers. He distinguishes between 'thin' descriptions, which embody unexamined and socially influenced preconceptions and refer to the internalisation and reproduction of expert knowledge; and 'thick' or 'rich' descriptions, which embody the personal meanings of the person involved, and are closer to the actuality of experience.

White and Epston draw on Bruner's[38] metaphor of 'landscape' to describe how narrative therapists can engage in conversations that range across landscapes of action (events in context over time) and landscapes of meaning (interpretations, values and meanings) and therefore enable the exploration of terrain which is known and familiar, as well as that which may be difficult or uncharted.

While there has been a growth of interest in narrative ideas across many disciplines, they have also attracted criticism which has particularly focused on the notion of narrative as having an important role to play in the way we think about identity. Strawson,[39] for example, challenges the claim that narrativity is 'a profound and universal insight into the human condition', and particularly contests the idea that we create the self through telling stories.

I offer a brief personal response here; see www.radcliffepublishing.com/devnarrativehcres/ for further discussion of Strawson's challenges.

NARRATIVE AS CREATING CONTINUITY

Clearly, I find narrative ideas about life and identity to be most useful in my thinking about the world and my own life. In the case of major life events such as illness, narrative is a means of making sense of 'peripeteia', of negotiating transitions and change, a way of mourning previous ways of being and of adjusting to different ways of being. In my own experience, the temporal and causal structure of narrative has provided a means of reflecting on the past in a way that has informed future choices, and made it possible for me to work with the illness stories of others. Thus it has enabled me to 'bridge the gap' between the 'me' I was before illness and the 'me' I am now, thereby creating continuity. We are temporal beings who live (and die) over a period of time. As Kearney[40] expresses it, 'Every human existence is a life in search of a narrative. This is not simply because it strives to discover a pattern to cope with the experience of chaos and confusion. It is also because each human life is always already an implicit story. Our very finitude constitutes us as human beings who, to put it baldly, are born at the beginning and die at the end' (p. 129). It is through narrative that we link events in time, making connections between our past, where we have come from, and our future, where we are heading. A sense of self thus depends on continuity even where there has been rupture, and such selfhood is created and recreated through the narrative process. Oliver Sacks[41] shows how, in the case of severe impairment of memory such as in Korsakov's syndrome, such continuity is lost, and with it goes our capacity to 'recollect the inner drama', the 'singular narrative, which is constructed unconsciously, by, through, and in us' (p. 105).

NARRATIVE AS CONSTITUTIVE OF SELF

In addition, the storytelling process has enabled the formation of new conceptions of self, thereby reflecting as well as restoring my sense of a coherent and unified life following disruption and change. Frank[42] uses the analogy 'narrative wreckage' (p. 53) to refer to the impact of illness on a person's life. He writes of illness stories carrying a sense of being 'ship-wrecked by the storm of the disease' (p. 54) and views storytelling as a way through this wreckage where 'a self is being formed in what is told' (p. 55). A small but nevertheless significant example of the way in which storytelling can be constitutive of self is when Pat talked of having 'been quite a feminine woman. I liked my high heels ... but I can't wear them any more'. The next time I saw her she said, 'I thought, why can't I wear my high heels? So I went out and bought a really high pair of sexy shoes!' It is through this narrative reconstruction of self, then, that we accommodate change, uncertainties and ambiguities. This is not done in isolation, however, but in dialogue and negotiation with others, and the selves they are becoming. Thus the narrative construction of self is relational and also social. 'Selfhood,' in Bruner's[43] words, 'involves a commitment to others as well as "being true to oneself"' (p. 69). The stories we tell do not belong to one person alone but are located within a community of interconnecting and involved others (family, friends, health care practitioners), as well as the broader, sociocultural setting.

AGENCY

As Bruner[44] expresses it, agency 'implies the conduct of action under the sway of intentional states' (p. 9). Identity formation involves interplay between personal agency, significant others and cultural reference points. In Bruner's[45] words, 'narrative acts of self-making are usually guided by unspoken, implicit cultural models of what selfhood should be, might be—and, of course, shouldn't be' (p. 65). The imagery used or encountered in illness is an example of the way in which such 'implicit cultural models' influence selfhood in illness (*see* Chapter Six.) In illness, narrative is a resource for negotiating disruption and major change, a means of making sense of the world and our lives in it. As agents, we act, and we do so for reasons—therefore we look for causal relationship between events.

EM Forster[46] defines plot as 'a narrative of events, the emphasis falling on causality' (p. 93). Plot represents significant interconnections rather than linear sequence and implies the question 'why?' In the novel, the plot is implicit—we expect 'every action, every word … to count' (p. 95). In real life, on the other hand, the question signifies the meaningful connections we make (or not) between events; it is certainly what we look for in contingencies such as serious illness, where our sense of agency is under threat. This 'intentionality' or meaning-seeking quality of being human is related to our capacity for reflexivity and is a distinctive feature of narrative. Narrative structure enables us to make sense of our lives and to find some kind of intelligibility in contingency. This is not to say that meaning can necessarily be found, but simply to say that we search for it. Serious illness teaches us that contingency and uncertainty are an inevitable and inescapable part of life.

NARRATIVE AND SUBJECTIVITIES

As the response of the nurse above demonstrates, narratives are a way of communicating subjectivities and inviting personal responses that have the potential to influence attitudes and practice, to bridge social divides and address issues of marginalisation in relation to illness and disability. Josselson and Lieblich[47] point to the 'transformational power of stories within societal organizations, and the use of stories as an agent of change' (p. xii). Narratives can act as a call to action in a personal sense but can also have a social and political role to play. The role of narrative in conveying the diversity of human experience in illness is recognised thus by Hurwitz *et al.*,[48] who assert:

> Human subjectivity should no longer be seen as the devalued opposite of scientific objectivity, linked in some zero-sum relationship whereby more of the one must necessarily mean less of the other. Rather, objective assessment (for example medical diagnosis) and objective intervention (for example, medical treatment or palliation) provide but one important dimension of knowing. However complete the objective dimension, if we exclude subjectivity and its narrative expression

through dialogue, we remove diversity of viewpoint and impoverish the knowledge we can gain about human suffering and the impact of our efforts to care. (pp. 3–4)

Science and life are nowhere more intimately connected than when illness or injury necessitates diagnosis, treatment and surgery. In an article entitled 'Neurology and the Soul', Sacks refers to 'a chasm between science and life, between the apparent poverty of scientific formulation and the manifest richness of phenomenal experience'[49] (p. 44). 'This chasm', he writes, 'is overwhelming in Biology in the study above all of mental processes and inner life, for these are unlike physical existence, distinguished by extreme complexity, unpredictability, and novelty; by inner principles of autonomy, identity and will … by a continuous becoming, evolution and development'.

The rise of the novel was a primary example of the capacity of narrative to convey subjectivities, or 'qualia'.[50,51] The complexity of first-person consciousness, or lived experience, and the difficulty in conveying it is expressed thus by Henry James:[52]

> Experience is never limited, and it is never complete; it is an immense sensibility, a kind of huge spiderweb of the finest silk threads suspended in the chamber of consciousness, and catching every airborne particle in its tissue. (p. 2)

There are various means by which we communicate such 'immense sensibilities'; art and music enable profound and complex expression. 'The inexpressible depth of music', as Schopenhauer wrote, 'so easy to understand and yet so inexplicable, is due to the fact that it reproduces all the emotions of our innermost being, but entirely without reality and remote from its pain …' (cited by Sacks[53] p. xi). The similarities between music and language have long been discussed.[54,55,56] The capacity of music to capture experience through its melody, rhythm, pitch and cadence is something I drew on in this research. However, language is one of the principal means by which we communicate personal subjectivities. As David Lodge[57] writes, 'Literature is a record of human consciousness, the richest and most comprehensive we have. Lyric poetry is arguably man's most successful effort to describe qualia. The novel is arguably man's most successful effort to describe the experience of individual human beings moving through space and time' (p. 10).

In my view, narrative is the principal form through which we structure subjective experience, whether in fiction or as a representation of 'real life'. In a paper about the role of narrative in research into lived experience, Bond[58] addresses the question of 'how we convey and deepen our understanding of lived experience' (p. 133) and the methodological and ethical challenges raised by the fact that lived experience is, 'by its very nature, both immediate and subjective' (p. 134). While he affirms the value and contribution of paradigms drawn from the natural sciences, he also recognises that 'rich personal accounts full of feelings, human relationships and personal backgrounds are transformed into impersonal conceptual frameworks in which thinking is privileged over action and emotion' (p. 133).

NARRATIVE INQUIRY

Narrative inquiry encompasses a broad range of approaches to research, which are based upon 'collecting, analysing, and re-presenting people's stories as told by them'[59] (p. 75). As Mishler[60] writes, 'Narrative research is an umbrella term that covers a large and diverse range of approaches, the result of a rapid expansion of this area of inquiry over the past dozen years' (p. xv).

Narrative inquiry, based on constructivist and social constructionist epistemologies, as well as on post-structural thinking, is well suited to an exploration of experience within a social and cultural context since it takes account of the place of knowledge and power in relation to individuals and society, and supplements the dominant narratives of medical discourse as well as those of popular culture through rich description that shows personal understandings and ways of living with illness and change. The representation of individual stories thus mediates between the personal and the social. In Bronwyn Davies'[61] words, 'The act of taking up and using language seems like an intensely personal experience but the effect shows how profoundly collective it is' (p. 34).

As I indicated in Chapter One, I was drawn to narrative because of its interdisciplinary nature, and its capacity to make sense of experience, in all of its personal, social and linguistic dimensions. However, formulated models such as Wengraf's[62] Biographic Narratives and semi-structured interview approach seemed to me to objectify contributors, and to lose something of the person in the process. I did not want a 'method' which viewed stories as data for analysis. This approach has its value, but it was not for me. I wanted to enter into relationship with my contributors' stories and to evolve a way of working which would be congruent with my values, and build on my existing skills and experience.

As a counsellor and counsellor educator, I had experience of facilitating and listening to stories, and of exploring meanings and understandings. McLeod[63] characterises the heart of qualitative research as 'doing one's utmost to map and explore the meaning of an area of human experience' (2001, viii), and suggests that many of the values, qualities and skills used in therapy are similar to those required in qualitative research, where we are seeking to elicit personal stories and to explore the life-world of a person in all its complexity and ambiguity.

Clearly, my thinking and curiosity about stories of illness and its impact on conceptions of self emerged from and were closely related to my own experience of illness and identity transformations. My initial research idea also had its origins in my background and theoretical orientation as a counsellor. My training was rooted in the person-centred approach of Carl Rogers,[64,65] and this had a strong influence on the way in which I worked with people, as the next chapter indicates.

REFLEXIVE SPACES

Such an approach requires a continual process of reflexivity through which a researcher reflects on her/his positioning, biases and assumptions.[66,67] Reflexivity, however, is a concept whose meanings are widely contested.[68]

As Speedy notes, 'reflexive styles'[69] (p. 42) are various and require different kinds of examination of researcher positioning. The extent to which the researcher is present in the text varies, as does the transparency with which positioning is acknowledged.

Writing conventions vary among and between academic genres; for example, discursive practice within the fields of counselling and psychotherapy differs according to theoretical orientation, and therefore concepts, and particular domains of language use associated with reflexivity signify different stances. Psychodynamic 'takes' on reflexivity, for example, might focus on issues of transference, countertransference and so on, whereas the humanistic or existential therapies take a more phenomenological stance, and emphasise therapists' authenticity, unconditional acceptance and empathy. McLeod notes that the development of writing traditions within each of the social sciences 'codifies its intrinsic values and philosophical assumptions'[70] (170).

Broadly speaking, and following Speedy,[71] I take reflexivity to refer to awareness and acknowledgement of the reflexive spaces between researchers and participants, researchers and texts, text and audience. The dynamics between each and all of these positions are complex and variable—arguably infinitely variable—for these reflexive spaces involve interplay between personal agency and various social and cultural domains of language use. Interplay between so many variables means that reflexive spaces are always dynamic rather than fixed. In relation to the research presented here, I regard these spaces as operating in three main spheres:

a. Within research conversations
b. Within the text in relation to issues of representation and analysis
c. Within the spaces between the text/performance and the audience

I take a position of embodied reflexivity, where my awareness and reflection on positioning is filtered through my subjectivities (while acknowledging that these are situated within different discursive practices) and therefore through relations of power/knowledge, or domains of language use. As Speedy expresses it, 'As soon as we enter this "space between us", we are entering relations of power. Reflexive/liminal spaces are, therefore, highly political, personal, imaginative and social spaces' (p. 28).

Decisions such as if and how researcher presence is shown within a text are undoubtedly ambiguous. I do not regard the presence of the authorial 'I' in a text as denoting a particular reflexive stance any more than the absence of 'I' denotes the neutrality of a text. While awareness and reflection on researcher subjectivity may contribute to the meanings implied by researcher-writer or inferred by audiences, all I can try to do is to be as aware as possible and as transparent as possible about my intentions and positioning; my stance of embodied reflexivity is therefore fluid and open to challenge, rather than fixed.

If researcher subjectivity tales place within discourses and the construction of selfhood emerges within contexts of social interaction, then the person 'I' am is relative to the domains of language use (or discursive practices) in which I engage. For example, within my research conversations I was positioned variously as fellow patient/researcher/co-researcher/co-participant/mother who has been lucky to see her children grow up, as well as counsellor/prospective author, and so on. As I write this, my identity claims as former patient, author, researcher and co-participant move in and out of view, depending on which claim I privilege. As McLeod[72] writes:

> On one hand, qualitative research is indeed personal, and the promotion and communication of the reflexive awareness of the expectations and experiences of the researcher contribute to the meaningfulness of a research report. On the other hand, the subjectivity of the researcher does not command a privileged position. Personal statements made by researchers are themselves positioned within discourses. (p. 201)

For example, in the information sheet I sent out to contributors, I referred to 'themes', thus taking for granted the discourses of qualitative research. In my first meeting with Jim, he questioned me as to what I meant by this—an important reminder to me of the assumptions I was making about shared understanding.

Frank[73] argues for the importance of reflexivity in countering a 'morality of distance' (p. 470). This has certainly been my own position, but as McLeod[74] notes, 'acknowledging the personal dimension of qualitative research, and knowing what to do about it, are two quite different things' (p. 195). For myself, this has meant an ongoing process of questioning and ethical decision-making, which has felt uncertain at times and close to the 'ambivalent practices of reflexivity' addressed by Davies *et al.*[75] I found it difficult to decide where and how to place myself in this text: I was unsure about placing my autoethnographic chapter as an introduction to this book, since I did not want my illness story to take precedence in any way over those of Pat, Jan, Jim and Yasmin. Yet it played a crucial role in this research; had I not been ill, I would have made very different choices in my life.

My illness experience has been fundamentally important in my relationships with participants; it was an important reference point in that it sensitised me to issues such as living with a heightened sense of mortality, and therefore it opened up spaces in relation to others' stories. It was the sharing of common ground such as the experience of vulnerability and loss of power and control, which allowed a degree of equality in those relationships. I regard myself as accountable to my participants, and while I still held power in the privileged position of researcher, I tried to hold that power in awareness. Nevertheless, the final decisions in terms of research practices and representation have been ultimately my responsibility. After considerable reflection, I decided to place my story at the beginning since it served as a context for the research and for the particular narrative methodology I developed. My positioning in relation to illness has been important in my relationships with contributors, and in the ways I have written their stories; to have situated myself as observer and 'outsider' would have been dishonest, created distance and obscured my role in the knowledge construction process. In talking with me and in contributing their stories to this book, people have entrusted me with their most vulnerable experiences, and therefore my capacity to access my own vulnerability has been vital, alongside keeping the focus of attention on their stories.

In the next chapter, I describe how the development of my approach to narrative research drew on the concepts and values outlined above. I describe my approach to 'data collection and analysis', or as I prefer to phrase it, research relationships and ethical stance, before examining how we might evaluate this type of approach to narrative inquiry.

REFERENCES

1. Damasio A. *The Feeling of What Happens: body and emotion in the making of consciousness.* London: Vintage; 1999.
2. Dennett D. *Consciousness Explained.* London: Penguin; 1991.
3. Polkinghorne DE. *Narrative Knowing and the Human Sciences.* Albany, NY: State University of New York; 1988.
4. Bruner J. *Actual Minds, Possible Worlds.* Cambridge, MA: Harvard University Press; 1986.
5. Bruner J. *Acts of Meaning.* Cambridge, MA: Harvard University Press; 1990.
6. Bruner J. *Making Stories: law, literature, life.* New York, NY: Farrar, Straus and Giroux; 2002.
7. Ibid.
8. Ibid.
9. Ibid.
10. Bruner, 1986, op cit.
11. Bruner, 2002, op cit.
12. McLeod J. *Narrative and Psychotherapy.* London: Sage; 1997.
13. Freedman J, Coombs G. *Narrative therapy: The social construction of preferred realities.* New York, NY: Norton; 1996.
14. McAdams DP. *The Stories We Live By: personal myths and the making of the self.* New York, NY: William Murrow; 1993.
15. Neisser U, Fivush R. *The Remembering Self: construction and accuracy in the self-narrative.* 1994 ed. New York, NY: Cambridge University Press; 1973.
16. White M, Epston D. *Narrative Means to Therapeutic Ends.* New York, NY: Norton; 1990.
17. Etherington K. *Trauma, the Body and Transformation.* London: Jessica Kingsley; 2003.
18. Frank A. *The Wounded Storyteller: body, illness and ethics.* Chicago, IL: University of Chicago Press; 1995.
19. Charon R. *Narrative Medicine: honoring the stories of illness.* Oxford: Oxford University Press; 2006a.

20. Murakami H. *Underground*. London: Vintage; 2003.
21. Buber M. *I and Thou*. Edinburgh: T&T Clark; 1937.
22. Davies B. *(In)scribing Body/Landscape Relations*. Walnut Creek, CA: Alta Mira Press; 2000a.
23. Ibid.
24. McLeod, op cit.
25. Gergen K. Therapeutic professions and the diffusion of deficit. *J Mind Behav.* 1990; **11**: 353–68.
26. McLeod, Foreword. In: Payne M. *Narrative Therapy: an introduction for counsellors*. London: Sage; 2002. p. ix.
27. White M, Epston D, op cit.
28. White M. *Re-authoring Lives: interviews and essays*. Adelaide: Dulwich Centre Publications; 1995.
29. White M. Reflecting team work as definitional ceremony re-visited. In: *Gecko: a journal of deconstruction and narrative ideas in therapeutic practice*. Adelaide: Dulwich Centre Publications; 1999.
30. White M. *Reflections on Narrative Practice: essays and interviews*. Adelaide: Dulwich Centre Publications; 2000.
31. White M. Re-engaging with history: the absent but implicit. In: White M, editor. *Reflections on Narrative Practice: essays and interviews*. Adelaide: Dulwich Centre Publications; 2000.
32. Foucault M. *Power/Knowledge: selected interviews and other writings*. Gordon C, editor. New York, NY: Pantheon Books; 1980.
33. White, Epston, op cit.
34. Lyotard JF. *The Postmodern Condition: a report on knowledge*. Bennington G, Massumi B, translators. Minneapolis, MN: University of Minnesota Press; 1979.
35. Gergen K. *An Invitation to Social Construction*. London: Sage; 1999.
36. Geertz C. *Local Knowledge: further essays in interpretive anthropology*. New York, NY: Basic Books; 1983.
37. Ryle G. *The Concept of Mind*. London: Hutchinson; 1949.
38. Bruner, 1986, op cit.
39. Strawson G. Against narrativity. *Ratio*. 2004b; **17**(4): 428–52. Epub 2004 Dec.
40. Kearney R. *On Stories*. London and New York, NY: Routledge; 2002.
41. Sacks O. *An Anthropologist on Mars*. London: Picador; 1995.
42. Frank, 1995, op cit.
43. Bruner, 2002, op cit.
44. Bruner, 1990, op cit.
45. Bruner, 2002, op cit.
46. Forster EM. *Aspects of the Novel*. London: Penguin; 1927.
47. Josselson R, Lieblich A, editors. *Making Meaning of Narratives, Vol. 6*. London: Sage; 1999.
48. Hurwitz B, Greenhalgh T, Skultans V, editors. *Narrative Research in Health and Illness*. London: BMJ Books; 2004.
49. Sacks O. Neurology and the soul. *New York Review of Books*. 1990 Nov 2.
50. Dennett, op cit.
51. Sacks, 1990, op cit.
52. James H. The art of fiction. In: *Partial Portraits*. New York, NY: Macmillan; 1888.

53. Sacks O. *Musicophilia*. London: Picador; 2007.

54. Ibid.

55. Gardner H. *Frames of Mind: the theory of multiple intelligences*. New York, NY: Basic Books; 1983.

56. Storr A. *Music and the Mind*. New York, NY: Free Press; 1992.

57. Lodge D. *Consciousness and the Novel*. London: Secker & Warburg; 2002.

58. Bond T. Naked narrative: real research? *Counselling and Psychotherapy Research (CPR)*. 2002; **2**(2): 133–8.

59. Etherington K. *Becoming a Reflexive Researcher: using our selves in research*. London: Jessica Kingsley; 2004.

60. Mishler EG. *Storylines: craft artists' narratives of identity*. Cambridge, MA: Harvard University Press; 1999.

61. Davies B, op cit.

62. Wengraf T. *Qualitative Research Interviewing: biographic narratives and semi-structured methods*. London: Sage; 2001.

63. McLeod J. *Qualitative Research in Counselling and Psychotherapy*. London: Sage; 2001.

64. Rogers CR. *On Becoming a Person*. Boston, MA: Houghton Mifflin; 1961.

65. Rogers CR. *A Way of Being*. Boston, MA: Houghton Mifflin; 1980.

66. Etherington, op cit.

67. Hertz R. *Reflexivity and Voice*. London: Sage; 1997

68. Speedy J. *Narrative Inquiry and Psychotherapy*. Basingstoke: Palgrave Macmillan; 2008.

69. Ibid.

70. McLeod J, op cit.

71. Speedy, op cit.

72. McLeod, 2001, op cit.

73. Frank A. The pedagogy of suffering: moral dimensions of psychological therapy and research with the ill. *Theory Psychol*. 1992; **2**: 467–85.

74. McLeod, 2001, op cit.

75. Davies B, Browne, Honan E, Laws C, *et al*. The ambivalent practices of reflexivity. In: *Qualitative Inquiry*. 2004; **10**(3): 360–89.

CHAPTER 9

From rationale to method: relationships, ethics and accountability

THE EVOLUTION OF MY RESEARCH METHODS

In the previous chapter, I explored the ideas and thinking that have informed my approach to research. In this chapter, I describe the development of an approach to narrative inquiry that draws on those underlying concepts. I do not offer a prescriptive method here that is clear and uncomplicated; rather, I show how the process was not simply a matter of the straightforward application of existing methods but one of evolution and adaptation to context and circumstances.

The development of interdisciplinary approaches to qualitative research has opened up possibilities for methodologies which blur the distinctions between the arts and the social sciences: innovative methodologies that can capture individual dimensions of experience and also take account of the relationship between personal agency and cultural context; collaborative and participatory approaches to research that can provide insight into sensitive and culturally complex issues. As the previous chapter shows, my approach to narrative inquiry has been informed by humanistic approaches to counselling and research alongside contemporary critical thinking based on social constructionist and poststructuralist ideas.

RESEARCH RELATIONSHIPS

Serious illness divides the sick from the well, and particularly the patient from the healthcare practitioner. It separates the sick from daily life and from the lives of friends and family, and from a previous sense of self when healthy. It reminds us all of our frailty, temporality and mortality, and carries with it profound and painful emotions. I believe it was fundamentally important for me to be aware of these divisions with regard to my relationships with those who contributed to this research.

Any research which addresses inequalities, sensitive interpersonal issues, profound fear and anxiety, the fragility of the body, emotions of embarrassment and shame, change in status, loss of power and control, and the inevitability of death requires respect, humility and accountability. I believe it was important for me to remain aware that illness is not something that only happens to others, but affects us all; we are all subject to the contingencies of health problems; we are all mortal. The development of trustworthiness within research relationships requires recognition of the inequalities illness can bring, as well as an awareness of the way health difficulties can affect us all. As Speedy[1] notes, 'ethical practice in narrative inquiry is a reciprocal and relational space' (p. 51). As well as dividing the sick from the healthy, illness and mortality unite us as fellow human beings.

Charon[2] suggests four main types of division in relation to illness and health: mortality, context, causality and emotions. She then identifies five features of a narrative approach to medicine/healthcare—temporality, singularity, causality/contingency, intersubjectivity and ethicality (p. 22)—which bridge these divides. She also suggests that the development of awareness and narrative competence in these dimensions would greatly enhance the effectiveness of care. It was certainly important for me to be aware of these divisions, and I would suggest that attunement to the polarised positioning of the sick and the well (and to issues of social marginalisation) can be applied more broadly to narrative research in general; the stories we tell of our lives are of contingent events over time told by a particular person in a relational space, with ethical implications. Therefore, narrative approaches to research are particularly suitable for addressing social inequalities in all spheres of life. It is to this particularly relational feature of narrative and its place in my methodology that I now turn.

Cooper and McLeod[3] have written in favour of pluralistic approaches to research in counselling and psychotherapy, in which there is an 'ethical commitment … to valuing Otherness'. Cooper suggests pluralism can be regarded as a form of humanistic-existential ethic in which there is 'a commitment to conceptualising and engaging with people in a deeply valuing and respectful way' (p. 11).

Many have written of overlaps between research 'interviews' and therapy, both in terms of the experience of being part of a research project as therapeutic, and also in terms of the qualities and skills a therapist may bring to research.[4,5,6,7,8,9,10,11,12] In keeping with my view of narrative as an intersubjective relational dimension of being human, I will outline here some of the ways in which my counselling background has informed my ways of working.

As a person-centred counsellor whose training and experience was firmly rooted in humanistic principles of connection, authenticity and 'meeting at relational depth',[13,14] I knew how effectively the qualities of empathy, congruence and unconditional positive regard, or 'core conditions' as Rogers[15,16] terms them, could enable the telling of stories and the expression of meanings and understandings. The person-centred approach is fundamentally based on the values of equality and dialogue in relationship, and is closely related to the ideas of Martin Buber.[17] This relational 'way of being',[18] founded on humanistic principles of respect and equality, takes a phenomenological approach to the person and emphasises the way in which subjective experience constitutes the reality of each human being by placing trust in the 'actualising tendency' and inner resources of the individual.[19,20,21] The person-centred approach is, ideologically, 'of its time' and therefore takes an essentialist view of the person—in so far as it pays little *explicit* attention to the ways in which subjectivities are embedded within cultural contexts; however, there is *implicit* acknowledgement that subjective realities are informed by the social contexts in which we live.

My intention to facilitate, and to understand as closely as I could, the richness and complexity of subjective experience therefore required the development of an approach that would enable the expression of first-person experience in all its complexity and multiplicity. My original research idea had been to work in a purely person-centred way to facilitate the telling of stories. Some years previously, Mearns and McLeod[22] (p. 372) had convincingly argued the case for the person-centred approach as a valid means of inductive social research, and regarded it as a 'philosophy of the person or attitude toward life that can be expressed in the research act' (p. 389). I will briefly outline the core conditions and how they informed my approach to the research relationship. I will also refer to these in my reflections on the implications of this research for healthcare and research (*see* Chapters Eleven and Twelve).

CORE CONDITIONS

The qualities of congruence, acceptance and empathy are interconnected ways of being, though I will look at each one separately with reference to its place in the research relationship. Congruence is the term used by Rogers to refer to the quality of genuineness or authenticity: the willingness on the part of the therapist to be aware of her own responses and to communicate these to the client when appropriate. The quality of 'unconditional positive regard', or acceptance, refers to the counsellor's warmth, respect and willingness for the client to be whatever s/he is at that moment, without judgment or condition, as a separate person. It involves respect for the other person's 'frame of reference' and consistent acceptance of every dimension of her/his experience.

The quality of empathy refers to a process of attempting to delicately step into another's shoes and to sense the world as they experience it. Rogers[23] expresses it thus:

> It means entering the private perceptual world of the other and becoming thoroughly at home in it. It involves being sensitive, moment by moment, to the changing felt meanings which flow in this other person, to the fear or rage or tenderness or confusion or whatever that he or she is experiencing. It means temporarily

living the other's life, moving about in it delicately without making judgments (p. 142).

Empathy also involves tentatively communicating and checking these understandings. Rogers stressed the need 'to sense the client's world *as if* [my italics] it were your own, but without ever losing that "as if" quality'[24] (p. 99). This refers to the importance of *not* making assumptions about another person's experience from within one's own frame of reference. While we may resonate with another's experience, the blurred edges of identifying and empathising are easy to cross, and in the space between self and other, there is always, in Derrida's[25] word, 'differ*a*nce'—a term that he coined to refer to the elusiveness of meaning, and subtlety of both differing from ('différer'), and deferring to (déférer).

Our appreciation of someone else's experience is *always* partial and uncertain; empathy involves being aware of differences alongside similarity, and a recognition of what Levinas[26] terms 'alterity', or otherness. For me as researcher, this required a disciplined, reflexive process in terms of the relationship between my own experience and its place in conversations with my contributors.

The empathic process of delicately sensing another person's 'frame of reference' has several effects. It is a mutual engagement in searching for meanings, and as such, reduces isolation; or, as Rogers[27] writes, 'dissolves alienation' (p. 151). Thus it is a key means of bridging the 'divides' between the sick and the well to which Charon[28] refers, and of enabling the telling of stories which might otherwise go untold. I see empathy as predicated on a sense of connection, and as intertwined with acceptance and authenticity. We cannot truly empathise with others if we are passing judgment, and empathy expressed without authenticity would not only sound hollow, it would *be* hollow and not ring true. When someone listens empathically, he or she becomes a companion in our search for meanings, and this can enable the exploration of understandings, the telling of stories that might have gone untold and the discovery of meanings that lie at the 'edge of awareness', to use Gendlin's[29,30] term. Thus, empathy can offer access to intuitive 'knowing' as well as explicit understanding; it can also enable the expression of unspoken experience as well as habitual, often-told stories—indeed, such empathy may enable access to meanings that White[31] (after Derrida) refers to as 'absent but implicit'.

A DIALOGIC AND RELATIONAL SPACE

My experience of the storytelling process is that it is, or can be, reciprocal, connective and life-affirming: it flows from what Martin Buber[32] terms the '*a priori* of relation' (p. 43). Buber's view of what it is to be human as relational is that we gain a sense of our own identity and authenticity through relationships. He distinguishes two primary attitudes characterise our existence in the world; he differentiates the monologic *I-It* way of being from the dialogic *I-Thou*.

The *I-It* way of being is one in which we relate to others as objects; in Buber's words, 'man stands before things but not over against them in the flow of mutual action. Now with the magnifying glass of peering observation, he bends over particulars and objectifies them, or with the field-glass of remote inspection he objectifies them and arranges them as scenery' (p. 36). The dialogic, *I-Thou* attitude, on the other hand, is when we relate as persons and risk something of ourselves. It means, as Buber says, 'confirming the other' and 'accepting the whole potentiality of the other'.

Mearns,[33] and Mearns and Cooper use the concept of 'relational depth' to refer to moments of connection and intimacy in the therapeutic encounter, which they describe as, 'a state of profound contact and engagement between two people, in which each person is fully real with the Other, and able to understand and value the Other's experiences at a high level'[34] (p. xii). I believe we can be equally open to such moments in the research relationship. While the research relationship clearly differs from the therapeutic encounter, there is a sense in which such meeting at relational depth is not only respectful and genuine, but is facilitative of the telling of stories and the discovery of alternative meanings.

These values fundamentally underpin my approach to research, and since one of my aims was to explore as sensitively and fully as possible the experience of my contributors, then the relational qualities above are not just an ethical commitment but also enable the telling of rich and complex stories. If I engage with another in authentic, equal partnership without judgment, if I maintain and communicate the attitude that the person is the authority in his or her own world, this will foster trust and encourage further exploration of experience. If I am willing to pay close attention to her/his subjective experience, and to check out my understandings of each person's frame of reference, then this will enable the telling of stories that often go untold: stories which go beyond the culturally sanctioned discourses of illness, social myths of heroism, of 'being positive', or 'not giving in', and give voice to alternative stories.

I came to realise that the fact that I had also experienced serious illness and my willingness to draw on that in these relationships was a vital dimension of the knowledge-construction process. This is an approach to narrative research in which the research relationships and process are regarded as part of the 'analysis', in that the stories which unfold are co-constructions of knowledge in their own right. Rather than setting out to gather material solely for the purpose of future 'analysis', interpretation, and drawing of conclusions, I was also intending to participate in a form of collaborative research which drew on the practices of narrative therapy practitioners White and Epston,[35] where the concern is to create space for the performance of alternative stories. These alternative stories, or counter-narratives, resist the dominant storylines and 'truths' of normalising discourses, and in them the storytelling process itself is regarded as potentially transformative. I reflect further on the dynamic and transformative nature of this learning process in Chapter Twelve.

RESEARCH CONVERSATIONS

From the outset, I viewed my meetings with the people contributing to this study as opportunities for telling stories, and as research *conversations* rather than 'interviews'. While there is significant literature on research 'interviewing', such as the formulated structured and semi-structured methods of Wengraf[36] or the protocols of Lieblich,[37] it felt important to me to risk something of myself and relate as a person, rather than follow an interview manual. The people whose stories are represented in this book are not just their illnesses, any more than I am defined solely by my illness or story. While the focus of my research was on illness, I did not want to relate to people in a way that could potentially be reductive. However, I was aware that the focus of our meetings on specific aspects of experience would require me to be more directive and topic-oriented than in a therapy relationship. In short, I was confident that I had the necessary qualities and skills, while also aware that I had much to learn. My learning was enhanced by consulting my participants; for example, when Pat noted that she experienced one of our early meetings as more like a counselling session, I realised that my empathic responses had, at times, been narrowing the focus of our conversation rather than opening up spaces where a range of stories might be told.

My challenge was to evolve a way of working that would be congruent with my values and existing skills but would also accommodate my developing awareness of narrative approaches to therapy. In this, I drew particularly on the work of White and Epston[38] and its development by Bird,[39,40] Etherington,[41,42,43,44] Payne[45] and Speedy.[46,47] I also drew on the work of Clandinin and Connelly[48] in education research, and found particularly helpful their three-dimensional construct of narrative inquiry as temporal, situated and contextualised within a personal-social continuum. My training in experiential, person-centred work had made me very careful about the use of questions which might be viewed as interrogatory, and I proceeded with caution—and increasing confidence—to adopt a more questioning stance to open up areas of conversation.

Following the metaphor of landscapes of action and landscapes of meaning borrowed from Bruner[49] by White and Epston,[50] my questions moved back and forth across those territories to explore events over time (landscapes of action), as well as meanings and values (landscapes of meaning). As Speedy[51] notes, this metaphor 'provides co-researchers with some useful tools for navigating difficult or uncharted terrain together, and with ways of bringing to mind events or the meaning given to them that might otherwise have been overlooked or left out of the story altogether' (p. 68).

SELECTION OF CONTRIBUTORS

The in-depth relational nature of the research meant that the number of contributors would be restricted. I had originally anticipated working with a total of six to eight participants, but the richness and complexity of the stories from my first two participants, Pat and Jan, was such that I realised that it would be better to work with fewer people, and to do so by engaging with them and with their stories at 'relational depth'.[52,53] The emphasis was therefore on quality of relationship rather than on quantity of participants. The exact number could not have been determined beforehand, but the four people who contribute to this research provided a breadth and diversity of experience and context, while also allowing sufficient space to enable me to represent the richness and detail of each person's experience. Selection was on the basis that people had experienced serious health problems and major surgery. Since the nature of the research methods demanded introspection and reflection, I accessed contributors through counselling contexts. In order to ensure anonymity, I do not give more precise contextual or identifying information.

ETHICAL ISSUES

The principles on which research ethics are based are similar to those of counselling: a commitment to participants' well-being, autonomy, fidelity, justice and self-respect.[54,55,56,57] The British Association of Counselling and Psychotherapy (BACP) recently produced guidelines[58] for researchers are based on ethics of trust and trustworthiness between the people involved. This shift from fixed to relational ethics is aimed at fostering a climate of negotiation and an ongoing process of discussion between researcher and researched. The emphasis is on a continuing *process* of what Bond[59] refers to as 'ethical mindfulness', which is based on 'an ethic of trust' in relationships between researchers and participants.[60,61,62,63,64] The notion of an ethically mindful methodology that involves respect, the development of trustworthiness, integrity, compassion and care, as well as the management of research processes such as data protection, recognises the ways in which researchers are accountable to the people whose lives we are researching. This accountability involves awareness of potential inequalities and includes responsibility to research participants, sensitivity to issues of privacy, informed consent, respect for a person's wish to withdraw and confidentiality.

ETHICAL MINDFULNESS

In accordance with this notion of ethical mindfulness, and with my values and commitment to relating as equally as possible, the research relationships in this project have been carefully and continually negotiated. I see myself as being accountable to each person whose story is represented here. Ethical decisions have been and continue to be made on an individual basis.

As McLeod[65] reminds us, participation in this kind of in-depth work can be experienced as 'intrusive and demanding' and may reconnect participants with material that is distressing. While there is potential (and evidence) for therapeutic benefits as part of the research process, it was vital that participants were given detailed information about what would be involved so that they could make as informed a decision as possible before they agreed to take part.[66,67,68,69,70]

Therefore, as part of the *process* of informed consent, participants were given detailed, written information about what the study would involve, as well as regular opportunities to discuss this. The first meeting was intended as an opportunity for discussion and questions about ethical issues or dilemmas that could arise through the research project and how these could be addressed. In addition, since such rich, qualitative information could make confidentiality and anonymity more difficult, it was important that this was an ongoing consultative process in which contributors were able to see and respond to representations of their material before any of it was released or published. Therefore, I consulted contributors throughout about their continued participation and involvement in this research.

AN ETHICS OF AESTHETICS

As part of my commitment to participants, I tried to represent their stories in such a way as to be truthful to experience, while also preserving anonymity and confidentiality. Therefore, I observed what I have termed 'ethics of aesthetics'[71] (p. 52), in which the modes of representation prioritise literary truth over literal truth. As Speedy[72] reminds us:

> Narrative ethics then, position us differently in relation to ethics of care, justice, accountability and so forth, not by telling the literal truth (which in the case of ethical dilemmas and issues may not be possible to tell) but ... by creating the space for us to imaginatively feel our way into the experiences described, whilst remaining accountable to the spirits and values of the original storytellers. (p. 52)

Thus with the intention of preserving such anonymity and confidentiality as requested, I aimed for the 'verisimilitude' of stories that are crafted in such a way as to provide the space for resonance in readers, with the intention of producing transformative research that will influence practice and make a difference to people's lives. For, as Bakan[73] advises, 'Narrative research, based on the real lives of people made public, converts what is private into public; can violate privacy and can cause mental, legal, social and financial hurt and harm' (p. 3). I have sought to represent the stories in this book in ways which respect the rights and wishes of participants, and that do justice to their stories. Like West,[74,48] I hope these stories 'leap from the page ... and paint pictures in readers' minds'. Massumi,[75] in his preface to the philosophical work of Deleuze and Guattari, suggests the reader approaches the text in a spirit of openness, and asks questions such as, 'Does it work?' The question 'does it work?' could equally be applied to narrative research and raises issues of validity and how we evaluate research texts.

EVALUATION AND QUESTIONS OF VALIDITY

The strong and pervasive influence of the positivist, scientific paradigm continues to influence assumptions about what constitutes 'proper', valid research. Within the natural sciences, validity has traditionally rested on criteria of objectivity, impartiality and generalisability. And since qualitative research within the social sciences developed out of the natural sciences, realist agendas, values and practices are still regarded by many as the main criteria by which research may be evaluated. However, realist approaches to research can de-contextualise participants, researchers and methodology, and operate in reductive ways. The development of creative research practices that blur the boundaries between the arts and social sciences (such as narrative inquiry, autoethnography, creative non-fiction, magical realism, performative social science) have challenged notions of validity with its meanings of objective evidence and absolute Truth.

Nevertheless, the question of what we bring to our readings of narrative research, and how we evaluate such research, is important. Polkinghorne[76] observes that 'different kinds of knowledge claims require different kinds of evidence and argument to convince readers that the claim is valid' (p. 474). Speedy[77] finds that in navigating the tensions of producing relevant research for different purposes, she is 'drawn towards different criteria at different moments,' but ultimately finds that 'the most compelling criterion is that of transformation and emancipation' (p. 57).

In relation to this particular research project, I am making claims about both the value of narrative as a methodology and also about the 'findings', or rather the representations, of the illness narratives I have collected. The validity of this research therefore rests on the degree to which the knowledge claims I am making about personal accounts of illness experience are justified by the research methods I have used, and by the stories as represented here. If, as Polkinghorne[78] asserts, 'narrative inquiry makes claims about the meanings which life events hold for people, and how people understand situations, others, and themselves' (p. 476), then I am claiming that the representations in this book show particular understandings and also perhaps illuminate more universal features of illness experience in ways which might influence practice within healthcare.

The in-depth qualitative nature of this research was such that the number of participants had to be restricted; my intention was to work in depth and detail with people's stories and to do justice to this complexity in my representation. Therefore, I was clearly not aiming for generalisability, but transferability. In the terms of Judith Okely,[79] I aimed to use the specificity of experience 'in order to contextualize and transcend it' (p. 2). Serious illness and major surgery can happen to any of us, at any life stage, and thus raise fundamental and universal human issues, such as those of loss, transition, disability and mortality. Transferability therefore requires both a consideration of which issues might be seen to be fundamental, universal and broadly applicable, and also requires researcher reflexivity, contextual information about the sociocultural background of the stories, and the means by which they were gathered.

I am claiming 'validity' in its etymological sense of 'strength' and impact. I see the question of validity in this project as being one of *meaning* in relation to three reference points: the participant, the researcher and the audience. The claims I am making are about the capacity of this research to represent the lived experience of serious illness or health problems that require surgery and hospitalisation, and the effect of these on people's lives. I am also making claims about my own positioning both in terms of the way in which I work with the people in this study, and in terms of the way I '*re*-present' their stories. The final point of reference against which this research may be evaluated is in terms of the 'audience' or readers of this text.

Speedy[80] (p. 56), drawing on the work of writers from many disciplines, suggests the following criteria by which we may evaluate narrative research. While not all of these suggestions below will be appropriate for all narrative research, they are offered by Speedy as potential criteria for supporting the reading of narrative research. These criteria are clearly negotiable; they offer guidelines for participants, researchers and audiences as to how narrative research might be evaluated. I follow Speedy's suggestions below, with a set of my own criteria which are specific to this particular narrative inquiry.

SOME CRITERIA TO SUPPORT READINGS OF CREATIVE NARRATIVE RESEARCH

Transparency	<ul><li>How did the author(s) come to write this text?</li><li>How was the information gathered?</li><li>Does the writer make the purposes, perspectives and positions that have informed the construction of the text available?</li></ul>
Trustworthiness	<ul><li>Does this text seem 'truthful'—a credible account of a cultural, social, individual or communal senses of the world?</li><li>Are claims to verisimilitude (truthfulness) and knowledge embedded in multiple criteria that address 'lived experience'?</li></ul>
Aesthetic merit	<ul><li>Does this text succeed aesthetically?</li><li>Does it use creative practices that open up the text and invite interpretive responses?</li><li>Is the text artistically shaped, satisfying and (above all) *not boring?* Does the writing make my heart sing?</li></ul>

Reflexivity	• Does this text include a sense of personal embodiment and/or cultural embeddedness on the part of the author(s)? Is this text partial, situated and contingent?
Accountability	• Which community's interests does this text represent? In what ways are researchers accountable to those people? Are ethical issues and issues of collaboration/participation and power relations discussed? • How is the space between researchers and researched navigated? • Does the contribution made outweigh the ethical dilemmas/pain for participants/writers and readers? Is the separation of private and public spheres transgressed?
Substantive and enduring contribution	• Does this contribute to our understanding of social/cultural life and what it means to be a human being? • Will this text endure and be of some lasting value in the field?
Impact and transformation	• Does this resonate with me? • Does this affect me emotionally/intellectually/spiritually/politically? • Does this generate new questions? • Move me to try new research practices? Move me to action? • Transgress taken-for granted assumptions? • Transform/make a difference? • Implement an emancipatory agenda?

PERSONAL CRITERIA

In addition to the criteria above, I include my personal reference points, which are inevitably partial and situated; the questions that I have tried to bear in mind with regard to this particular project are concerned with *meaning* in relation to the following referents:

- **The participant**
  — Does the participant feel able to tell her or his story openly and without fear of judgment?
  — Does s/he feel accepted and understood?

— Does s/he feel related to 'as a person' and on equal terms?

— Does s/he trust this researcher?

— Can s/he explore and express complexity and multiplicity of meanings?

— Does s/he feel able to tell ambiguous or contradictory stories if s/he wishes to do so?

— Does s/he feel able to say 'no, I don't wish to talk about that aspect of my experience'?

— Does s/he feel able to withdraw from this research study if s/he wishes to do so?

— How do the written representations in this thesis or elsewhere correspond to her/his lived experience as s/he sees it?

— Does the writing reflect the multi-dimensional, multi-vocal complexity of experience? Does s/he recognise herself in the text? Does it capture the 'felt-sense' of experience?

- **The researcher**
  — Am I committed to relating as equally as possible?

  — Do I relate with compassion and humanity?

  — Am I genuine, accepting and empathic?

  — Am I willing to engage at relational depth?

  — Am I rigorous in monitoring my positioning within the research conversations, as well as interrogating my epistemological and ontological assumptions?

  — Do I extend this reflexivity to my analysis?

  — Does my analysis show evidence of reflection and critical thinking? Is it evocative and also intellectually challenging?

- **The audience**
  — Does the relationship between researcher and participant adequately facilitate the expression and exploration of complex experience? Is there sufficient information and transparency about the research relationships for the audience/reader to judge this?

  — Does the text invite the reader/audience into the participants' experience?

  — Does it evoke resonance, thoughts, personal stories, ideas in the reader?

  — Does it feel authentic?

  — Does it give sufficient information about the sociocultural context of these stories? Does it convince the reader that the research methods were appropriate to the claims made for authenticity?

  — Does it take a sufficiently reflexive stance in terms of researcher positioning and 'describe ways in which his or her own background experiences produced understandings through interaction with the text'[81] (p. 478)?

As Polkinghorne[82] reminds us, 'Validity is not inherent in a claim but is a characteristic given to a claim by the ones to whom the claim is addressed' (p. 474). Validity therefore is a question of intersubjective evaluation between the contributors, the researcher and the reader, and asks of the audience, 'Does this offer you what I claim it offers?' Thus it is my task to honour my contributors' stories and to convince the reader to enter into relationship with these stories as part of the validation process. In the following chapter, I unpack these questions of validity and evaluation further by addressing issues of representation and the approaches I have taken to writing and analysis.

REFERENCES

1. Speedy J. *Narrative Inquiry and Psychotherapy.* Basingstoke: Palgrave Macmillan; 2008.
2. Charon R. *Narrative Medicine: honoring the stories of illness.* Oxford: Oxford University Press; 2006a.
3. Cooper M, McLeod J. A pluralistic framework for counselling and psychotherapy: implications for research. *Counselling and Psychotherapy Research (CPR).* 2007; 7(3): 135–43.
4. Etherington K. The counsellor as researcher: boundary issues and critical dilemmas. *Br J Guid Counsell.* 1996; 24: 339–46.
5. Etherington K. Research with ex-clients: an extension and celebration of the therapeutic process. *Br J Guid Counsell.* 2001; 29(1): 5–19.
6. Etherington K. Life story research: a relevant methodology for counsellors and psychotherapists. *Counsell Psychother Res J.* 2009; 9(4): 225–33.
7. Hart N, Crawford-Wright A. Research as therapy, therapy as research: ethical dilemmas in new-paradigm research. *Br J Guid Counsell.* 1999; 27(2): 205–14.
8. Rosenthal G. The healing effects of storytelling on the conditions of curative storytelling in the context of research. *Qualitative Inquiry.* 2003; 9(6): 895–915.
9. Wosket V. *The Therapeutic Use of the Self: counselling, practice, research and supervision.* London: Routledge; 1999.
10. Kvale S. The psychoanalytic interview as qualitative research. *Qualitative Inquiry.* 1999; 5(1): 87–113.
11. McLeod J. *Doing Counselling Research.* London: Sage; 1994.
12. McLeod J. *Qualitative Research in Counselling and Psychotherapy.* London: Sage; 2001.
13. Mearns D, Thorne B. *Person-Centred Therapy Today.* London: Sage; 2000.
14. Mearns D, Cooper M. *Working at Relational Depth in Counselling and Psychotherapy.* London: Sage; 2005.
15. Rogers CR. *On Becoming a Person.* Boston, MA: Houghton Mifflin; 1961.
16. Rogers CR. *A Way of Being.* Boston, MA: Houghton Mifflin; 1980.
17. Buber M. *I and Thou.* Edinburgh: T&T Clark; 1937.
18. Rogers, 1980, op cit.
19. Ibid.
20. Thorne B. *Carl Rogers.* London: Sage; 1992. pp. 26–9.
21. Mearns D, Thorne B. *Person-Centred Counselling in Action.* London: Sage; 1988.
22. Mearns D, McLeod J. A person-centred approach to research. In: Levant R, Schlien J, editors. *Client-Centred Therapy and the Person-Centred Approach: new directions in theory, research and practice.* New York, NY: Praeger; 1984.
23. Rogers, 1980, op cit.

24. Mearns D, McLeod J, op cit.
25. Derrida J. *Writing and Difference*. Chicago, IL: University of Chicago Press; 1978.
26. Levinas E. *Otherwise than Being: or beyond essence*. Dordrecht, Boston, MA and London: Kluwer; 1991.
27. Rogers, 1980, op cit.
28. Charon, op cit.
29. Gendlin E. *Focusing*. New York, NY: Everest House; 1978.
30. Gendlin E. The client's client: the edge of awareness. In: Levant R, Schlien J, editors. *Client-Centred Therapy and the Person-Centred Approach: new directions in theory, research and practice*. New York, NY: Praeger; 1984. pp. 76–10.
31. White M. Re-Engaging with history: the absent but implicit. In: White, M, editor. *Reflections on Narrative Practice: essays and interviews*. Adelaide: Dulwich Centre Publications; 2000.
32. Buber, op cit.
33. Mearns, Thorne, op cit.
34. Mearns, Cooper, op cit.
35. White M, Epston D. *Narrative Means to Therapeutic Ends*. New York, NY: Norton; 1990.
36. Wengraf T. *Qualitative Research Interviewing: biographic narratives and semi-structured methods*. London: Sage; 2001.
37. Lieblich A, Tuval-Mashiach R, Zilber T, editors. *Narrative Research: reading, analysis and interpretation*. Thousand Oaks, CA: Sage; 1998.
38. White, Epston, op cit.
39. Bird J. *The Heart's Narrative: therapy and navigating life's contradictions*. Auckland, New Zealand: Edge Press; 2000.
40. Bird J. *Talk That Sings: therapy in a new linguistic key*. Auckland, New Zealand: Edge Press; 2004.
41. Etherington K. *Narrative Approaches to Working with Male Survivors of Sexual Abuse: the clients', the counsellor's and the researcher's story*. London: Jessica Kingsley; 2000.
42. Etherington K. *Trauma, the Body and Transformation*. London: Jessica Kingsley; 2003.
43. Etherington K. *Becoming a Reflexive Researcher: using our selves in research*. London: Jessica Kingsley; 2004.
44. Etherington K. *Trauma, Drug Misuse and Transforming Identities*. London: Jessica Kingsley; 2008a.
45. Payne M. *Narrative Therapy: an introduction for counsellors*. London: Sage; 2002.
46. Speedy, op cit.
47. Speedy J. The 'storied' helper: an introduction to narrative ideas in counselling and psychotherapy. *Eur J Psychother Counsell Health*. 2000; 3(3): 361–75.
48. Clandinin J, Connelly FM. *Narrative Inquiry: experience and story in qualitative research*. San Francisco: Jossey-Bass; 2000.
49. Bruner J. *Actual Minds, Possible Worlds*. Cambridge, MA: Harvard University Press; 1986.
50. White, Epston, op cit.
51. Speedy, 2008, op cit.
52. Mearns, Thorne, op cit.
53. Mearns, Cooper, op cit.

54. Bond, T. Codes of ethics and guidelines. In: Feltham C, Horton I, editors. *Handbook of Counselling*. London: Sage Publications; 2000.

55. Bond T. A question of trust: an introduction to the ethical guidelines for researching counselling and psychotherapy. *Counsell Psychother Res J*. 2004a; **4**(2): 4–9.

56. Bond T. Ethical guidelines for researching counselling and psychotherapy. 2004b; *Counsell Psychother Res J*. **4**(2): 10–19.

57. British Association for Counselling and Psychotherapy. *Ethical Framework for Good Practice in Counselling and Psychotherapy 2009*. Available at: www.bacp.co.uk. (Accessed 2009.)

58. Ibid.

59. Bond, 2000, op cit.

60. Bond, 2004a, op cit.

61. British Association for Counselling and Psychotherapy, op cit.

62. Bond, T. Intimacy, risk, and reciprocity in psychotherapy: intricate ethical challenges. *Transactional Analysis Journal*. 2006; **36**(2), 77–89.

63. Grafanaki S. How research can change the researcher: the need for sensitivity, flexibility and ethical boundaries in conducting qualitative research in counselling/psychotherapy. *Br J Guid Counsell*. 1996; **24**, 329–38.

64. Etherington K. Ethical research in reflexive relationships. *Qualitative Inquiry*. 2007; **13**(5); 599–616.

65. McLeod, 1994, op cit.

66. Rosenthal, op cit.

67. Wosket, op cit.

68. Kvale, op cit.

69. McLeod, 1994, op cit.

70. McLeod, 2001, op cit.

71. Martin V. Dialogue in the narrative process. *J Med Ethics*. **33**: 49–54.

72. Speedy, 2008, op cit.

73. Bakan D. *The Duality of Human Existence: isolation and communion in Western man*. Boston, MA: Beacon Press; 1966.

74. West D. DEAF-HEARING family life [PhD thesis]. University of Bristol, UK; 2009.

75. Massumi B. Translator's Foreword: pleasures of philosophy. In: Deleuze G, Guattari F. *A thousand plateaus*. London: Athlone Press; 1987.

76. Polkinghorne DE. Validity issues in narrative research. *Qualitative Inquiry*. 2007; **13**(4): 471–86.

77. Speedy, 2008, op cit.

78. Polkinghorne, op cit.

79. Okely J. Anthropology and autobiography: participatory experience and embodied knowledge. In: Okely J, Calloway H, editors. *ASA Monographs 29: Anthropology and Autobiography*. London and NY: Routledge; 1992.

80. Speedy, 2008, op cit.

81. Polkinghorne, op cit.

82. Polkinghorne, op cit.

CHAPTER 10

Representation

INTRODUCTION

As Bruner[1] notes (p. 23), 'Meaning always involves translation': in this chapter, I focus on the processes of translation from recorded research conversations, through to transcription, and to the representations in Chapters Two to Seven. While meaning involves translating experience into language, it is not, however, conveyed through words alone, but through the context and discourses in which a story is narrated and the intentions of speaker or writer. And since every encounter between speaker and listener (or text and reader) is potentially different, then meaning is always intersubjective and, in Iser's terms, indeterminate. He writes of the gaps in literary texts as 'enabling us to recreate the world it presents ... This virtual dimension is not the text itself, nor is it the imagination of the reader: it is the coming together of text and imagination'.[2] (p. 284) Therefore, such translation, whether as literary narrative or speech act, is part of a dialogue between text and audience in which the latter perceives and actively contributes to the text; the discourse of the text, as Bruner[3] puts it, 'recruit[s] the reader's imagination' (p. 25). In phenomenological terms, meaning making takes place when consciousness engages with objects in the world. It is our capacity as 'intentional' human beings to engage interactively and dynamically in constructing meaning and making sense of the world.

In medicine, such representation takes the form of clinical notes, or the case report. Rita Charon[4] has developed a narrative approach to representation which takes the form of personal, reflective writing that complements her clinical notes. This is in the form of a 'parallel chart', which is a narrative account of a clinical encounter with a patient that enables the practitioner to 'dwell in that patient's presence' and to 'grasp the significance of actions, words, or feelings' (p. 149).

TRANSCRIPTION AS INDWELLING

Polanyi[5,6] uses the term 'indwelling' to refer to the immersion of oneself in the material or data in question: 'indwelling' refers to an intuitive knowing or being in experience as opposed to observing or interpreting data. The depth and quality of my relationships with participants and with their material was such that I decided to prioritise this process of 'indwelling' both in terms of the way in which I engaged in our research conversations, and also in the process of transcription and representation, which I set out below.

In translating the stories into transcribed conversations, I made choices about whether or not to represent pauses, intonation, pitch and timbre. Over time, I evolved a way of working which enabled me to be as 'in tune' with my contributors' stories as I could. My own difficulties in typing with my non-dominant hand meant that the transcription process took a very long time. However, I was reluctant to hand over recordings of our conversations to someone else for transcription; this was partly because I felt the unique voice of each person carried a sense of embodied presence in all its particularity and multiplicity. Thus, asking someone else to listen to the recordings felt to me as if I was removing a layer of anonymity from a contributor. In addition, I felt I was less likely than another transcriber to mishear each contributor's actual words since I had been part of the conversation. I had the idea of speaking my contributors' stories out loud, recording these and then employing someone to help with transcription. I found this process of indwelling to be a valuable means of tuning in to the voice of each contributor, with its particular timbre, inflection, intonation and personal language, and this helped me to reconnect with each person as I immersed myself in the recordings.

FROM TRANSCRIPTION TO NARRATIVE WRITING

The next stage of translation was from the recorded and transcribed conversations into the representations such as those in this book. In this intersubjective configuration, I moved from the contributors' stories as told in our meetings, to dwelling in those stories, and to their representation. This embodied process of dwelling in a sense of each person's presence and of writing her/his story enabled the discovery of the many facets and dimensions of experience. The intersubjective mediation and translation combined, in Charon's[7] words, 'complex processes of perception, neural handling, accruing of associated impressions, and then imaginative filling out, *developing* that which is seen into something created anew' (p. 140).

While I can never fully *know* the subjective experiences of Pat, Jan, Jim and Yasmin, and while my listening and representation are inevitably filtered through my perceptions and frames of reference, my responsibility *and* accountability to each person was to remain as close as possible to his/her story in the representations I was to create. While my contributors had, and indeed still have, the option of reading and responding to my representations should they wish to do so, in the end the responsibility for this is mine. It has been an act of faith on their part to allow me this licence. This has been a particular responsibility with regard to Yasmin, who died in the course of the research, and was unable to see the later stages of my 'representation' of her story.

REPRESENTATION AND PERFORMATIVITY

The movement between research conversations, interpretations and representations is analogous to a musical performance in which the musician brings interpretive capacities to the composition in order to capture the music and convey some sense of its spirit and meaning. Mishler[8] uses such a musical analogy to compare interpretation of transcripts to the performance of music from a score:

> Translating a score into music, a task similar to that of interpreting speech from a transcript, requires a competent performer, or mastery of the medium that permits 'filling in' gaps in the score in order to "make" music. (p. 34)

My role of 'mediating' between our actual research conversations, transcriptions and representations in this book can be likened to that of an actor or musician whose task is to engage with the feelings and meanings of composers or playwrights, and to bring their work to life through performance. In my re-creations and re-configurations of the contributors' stories, I have similarly aimed to bring experience to life on the page; in that sense I had the privilege and responsibility of 'performing' the stories of Pat, Jan, Jim and Yasmin to an 'audience'. If the 'performance' 'works' for someone, then it does so in the space between self and other, through moments of connection and resonance.

Writing on musical creation and re-creation, cultural theorist Edward Said[9] suggests, 'The best interpreters of poetry and music allow both their audience and themselves … the proposition that the work being presented is *as if* created by the performer … so performance of a work of music aims at identity: between interpretation and the work, between performer and listener, between this particular work and other works, and so forth' (p. 89). This is reminiscent of Rogers' conceptualisation of empathy, in which we allow personal resonance and recognition to infuse our responses while retaining an *as if* quality, and an awareness of the other person's frame of reference. Thus paradoxically we hold in awareness both similarity and difference. In representing my contributors' stories, I felt a moral imperative to do so in such a way as to convey their meanings, intentions and aspirations in participating in this study.

Pelias[10] argues in favour of the methodological power of performative writing on the grounds that it 'expands the notion of what constitutes disciplinary knowledge' (p. 417) and is a style of scholarship that is just as rhetorical as paradigmatic formal argument. While performative writing features the complexity of lived experience, it does so not indiscriminately, but by selection and shaping, with a view to evoking experience as opposed to recording it. It is, Pelias writes:

> … both an evocation of human experience and an enabling fiction. Its power is in its ability to tell the story of human experience, a story that can be trusted and a story that can be used. It opens the doors to a place where the raw and the

genuine find their articulation through form, through poetic expression, through art'. (p. 418)

Performative writing can open up space for personal resonance and engage imagination, hearts and minds. By acknowledging representation as partial, contextualised and positioned, and by valuing 'the fragmentary, the uncertain', performative writing can create 'a space where others might see themselves'[11] (p. 419) and inspire critical reflection on life experience, constructions of self and relationships within sociocultural contexts. I aspire to 'performative writing', which acknowledges complexity and invites engagement on many levels—intellectual and affective, narrative and paradigmatic, personal, social, spiritual and political.

Becker[12] describes narrative as 'the performance of bodily experience' and as a way of gaining 'access to bodily distress' (p. 14). It was with the intention of conveying such embodied distress that I chose to represent my contributors' narratives by means which included a form of creative non-fiction and poetic expression. In using these modes of representation, which I outline in more detail below, I selected and shaped material from research conversations that were themselves 'performances' of bodily experience in illness. Indeed, Mattingly[13] conceptualises clinical encounters as potential 'healing dramas' and demonstrates how such 'performed narratives can play a powerful role in clinical care' (p. 74). I similarly view the narratives of Pat, Jan, Jim and Yasmin as performative at each stage of the telling: as first told to me, in the retellings, and in representations at conferences or for publication. Therefore, as 'healing dramas', they have the potential to contribute to and change practice.

DATA ANALYSIS: THE SPECIFICS OF REPRESENTATION

A key issue in narrative research is whether stories are regarded as knowledge in their own right or as raw material or data for subsequent analysis. Polkinghorne[14] makes the distinction between *narrative analysis* and *analysis of narratives*: narrative analysis regards stories as knowledge *per se*, which, as Etherington[15] writes, 'constitute the social reality of the narrator' (p. 81); however, according to Polkinghorne, analysis of narrative treats narratives as 'raw' data through which to 'locate common themes or conceptual manifestations' (p. 13). (For further discussion and examples, *see* Etherington.[16,17,18,19])

I draw on both approaches to material and use forms of what might be termed 'literary analysis': I *re*-present material in ways that blur these distinctions, and draw on literary approaches to research (*see* Etherington,[20,21,22,23] Clough,[24] Ellis,[25,26,27] Frank,[28] Richardson,[29,30,31,32,33,34] Sparkes[35] and Speedy[36]).

The stories as represented in Part One are intended (as a form of 'narrative analysis') to convey a sense of each person's experience in its depth, richness and texture; here, my intention was to create a coherent story, to ensure 'space' for the voice of each storyteller, and to retain something of the integrity of the story as it unfolded in dialogue with me. Frank[37] writes of 'thinking with' stories as something we do when we enter another's story and allow our 'own thoughts to adopt the story's immanent causality, its temporality and its narrative tensions' (p. 158); I crafted the stories in a way that, I hoped, would facilitate this personal engagement.

However, as Leach notes, the 'relentless forward linearity' of narrative, with its dominant tropes of life as a journey, may have limitations as a metaphor of experience: as Leach[38] writes, 'Stories can go in many directions. They circle and backtrack, they double back on themselves like hypertexts, they wander down side paths, one story is passed on from person to person' (p. 19). In addition, some experiences may not be readily storied; they may exceed our vocabulary or understanding; they may be chaotic or contradictory, for as Edward Bruner[39] puts it, 'life experience is richer than discourse'. However, narrative thinking need not be confined to a linear sequential form: stories can be suggested more obliquely through the use of metaphor, or in Bird's[40] phrase, 'talk that sings' and 'brings us closer to the experience of poetry' (p. 30). Therefore in both the 'narrative analysis' chapters and the thematic 'analysis of narrative' sections, I represent my contributors' stories by drawing on devices such as poetry and on a form of creative non-fiction.

CREATIVE NON-FICTION

My approach to representing the stories in Part One developed out of my own experience of writing.[41,42,43] In *Out of my Head*, I set out to recreate and evoke the subjective reality of my illness in such a way as to draw the reader into my world as I had experienced it at that time, with all its inherent tensions and uncertainties. In order to do this, I drew on the narrative devices of the non-fiction novel used by writers such as Truman Capote,[44] Hunter S Thompson,[45] and Tom Wolfe,[46] where techniques such as the use of dialogue, rich description and scene-setting engage the reader. In a discussion of Wolfe's 'New Journalism', literary theorist David Lodge[47] describes how Wolfe used such novelistic strategies to 'generate an excitement, intensity and emotive power'. According to Lodge,[48] the 'non-fiction', or biographical novel, 'takes a real person and their real history as the subject matter for imaginative exploration, using the novel's techniques for representing subjectivity rather than the objective evidence-based discourse of biography' (p. 4). In his introduction to *The New Journalism*, Wolfe[49] describes the progress of the genre through the 1960s and how it was based on four literary devices: telling the story by creating scenes rather than summarising; telling the story through the consciousness of a particular person and in a way which 'gives the reader the feeling of being inside the character's mind and experiencing the emotional reality of the scene as he experiences it' (p. 46); giving sufficient description and detail to evoke a particular setting; and using dialogue rather than reported speech. Realistic dialogue, according to Wolfe, 'establishes and defines character more quickly and effectively than any other single device' (p. 46).

While my book was an account of my experience written entirely from my perspective (*see* Chapter One), my representations of the stories in Chapters Two to Five (though clearly filtered through my consciousness) were crafted to focus primarily on each person's story as it was constructed in our conversations. In writing these chapters, I used a form of 'creative non-fiction' through which I tried to 'show' rather than 'tell'.[50,51] I aimed to do this in a manner that I hoped would convey the immediacy and particularities of experience and invite the reader to engage with Jan, Jim, Pat and Yasmin as people, as well as reflect on the issues their stories raise. In recreating their stories, I selected dialogue from our research conversations, which I then shaped to give focus: an editing and crafting process intended to give the stories a narrative structure that would work 'on the page'. My intention was also to be transparent about process and to exemplify method as well as content. As Speedy,[52] from the perspective of 'collaborative co-inquirer', observes, 'Quite a number of researchers would benefit from more 'showing' what happens in narrative research conversations' (p. 61). What I have attempted to do here is to show a particular approach to research conversations. I do not present this as in any way definitive or prescriptive, but rather as an approach that evolved within the context and parameters of this particular narrative inquiry.

While I was reluctant to approach the stories of those with whom I work in a reductive way, I was aware that I wished to represent my research with a critical edge that would enhance its representational power and analytical force. For conference presentations, I focused on particular areas of experience such as isolation, transformation or professional identity and selected relevant speech from our conversations. For my thesis and for Part One of this book, I set out to tell the stories in a more self-contained way.

So, to summarise, my use of creative non-fiction was intended to:

- Focus on experience through selecting the detail from our research conversations
- Be transparent about the ways in which the stories were shaped through dialogue and co-construction; the relational nature of our research conversations
- Tell the stories in terms of events and meanings (Bruner's landscapes of action and consciousness')[53]
- Offer some interpretive reflection on the meanings within the story
- Provide a reflexive layer with regard to my own positioning, while keeping the focus on each person

POETRY

The representation of material from research interviews and conversations in poetic form has become increasingly popular within human sciences such as ethnography and counselling/psychotherapy. The use of stanzas (*see*, e.g. Gee,[54,55] McLeod and Balamoutsou,[56] Richardson,[57,58,59,60,61,62] and Etherington[63,64,65]) can effectively represent the rhythms, pauses and cadence of spoken language. For example, Jan describes her very early memories of hospital as 'not the usual memories' but of 'sensory things'; the stanza form seemed to me to capture the impressionistic nature of those memories and to represent her pauses and pace as she drifted back in time and traced the immediacy of those early sensory impressions (sights, sounds and smells). Poetic form can offer researchers a powerful and evocative means of distilling and capturing experiential memory which lies at the edges of language. Shotter[66] draws our attention to poetic forms of talk that 'first "strike" us or "arrest" us; they put reality, so to speak, on "freeze-frame" and "move" us to search that freeze-frame for ways in which to relate ourselves responsively to aspects of it' (p. 86).

However, while the stanza can be used to produce text which evokes the pauses, silence and emphasis of speech, it does not of itself make 'poetry'. As Richardson[67] (p. 882) neatly reminds us:

> A line
> break does
> not
> a poem
> make.

I found this a very useful reminder when I first tried out poetic representation; breaking up speech by using line breaks does not necessarily enhance its impact, nor constitute poetry. While the poetic *form* may be closer to speech than prose, poetry—whether free verse or traditional—is *crafted*. Nevertheless, bearing in mind Denzin's[68] point that 'good ethnography always uses language poetically and good poetry always brings a situation alive in the mind of the reader' (p. 26), poetic form can offer a powerful means of capturing and conveying experience in all its ambiguity, paradox and complexity. By enhancing the impact of representation and analysis, it can be, as Richardson[69] claims, 'a viable method for seeing beyond social scientific conventions and discursive practices' (p. 877).

Practices of 'writing as inquiry' and poetic representation such as those of Richardson[70,71,72,73,74,75] and Cixous[76] can also open up creative and analytic possibilities. Cixous in particular regards the poetic qualities of language as a means of discovery and 'reaching towards a place where knowing and not-knowing touch' (p. 38). I have also found poetry can open up a space where I may discover meanings that lie at the edge of my awareness; indeed it was the writing of the poem 'Raging Torrent'[77] (included in Chapter One) that enabled me to realise that writing is not only representational but is a means and process of discovery and transformation. In Chapter Six, I draw on this more creative use of poetic form as one of the ways in which I explore the use of imagery in the stories in this book.

Arthur Frank[78] writes of 'thinking with' stories as an act of engagement and empathy, and describes this as a 'fundamental moral act' (p. 25). I believe the representation of another person's stories is a similar moral act; a responsibility to represent experience in a way that is respectful, relational and engaging, and which resists what Raymond Williams[79] refers to as the 'immediate and regular conversion of experience into finished products', where 'relationships, institutions, formations in which we are still actively involved are converted into … formed wholes rather than forming and formative processes' (p. 128). This opposition to 'fixed forms' (p. 129), reminiscent of Carl Rogers'[80] conceptualisation of empathy as a *process* of 'being sensitive moment by moment to the changing felt meanings which flow in another person' (p. 142), seems to me to be in accord with a literary representation of experience and meanings as evolving through interaction and engagement, and through negotiating the tensions between voice(s), signature and audience (*see* Clandinin and Connelly,[81] p. 149).

While under no illusions as to my need to work on and develop my literary abilities, my aspiration is to portray stories that touch the hearts of an audience in the way that they touched my heart when I participated in these research conversations. Therefore I have tried to *re*-present the stories with the hope of 'transporting' the reader of the text as my contributors and I tell stories of illness and negotiate the 'twists and turns' of shifting identities. Pelias' 'methodology of the heart',[82] Ellis' 'heartful' ethnography,[83] and Sandelowski's 'appeal to the heart'[84] seem to me to offer ways to be close to the spirits and intentions of the storytellers. As Sandelowski puts it:

> The proof for you is in the things I have made, how they look to your mind's eye, whether they satisfy your sense of style and craftsmanship, whether you believe them and whether they appeal to your heart. (p. 61)

My hope is that these stories will appeal to hearts and minds and, in some small way, 'spiral towards actual change in the world'[85] (p. 138). In the final chapters of the book, I suggest some of the ways in which this research might be relevant in the field of healthcare. In Chapter Eleven, I consider some of the implications for healthcare education and practice. In Chapter Twelve, I draw the book to a close, with some reflections on what I have learnt as I have made the transition from counsellor to researcher. In my closing reflections, I return to my autoethnographic voice.

REFERENCES

1. Bruner J. *Actual Minds, Possible Worlds*. Cambridge, MA: Harvard University Press; 1986.
2. Iser W. The Reading Process: a phenomenological approach. *New Literary History*. 1972; 3(2): 279–99.

3. Bruner, op cit.
4. Charon R. *Narrative Medicine: honoring the stories of illness.* Oxford: Oxford University Press; 2006a.
5. Polanyi M. *Personal Knowledge: towards a post-critical philosophy.* Chicago, IL: Chicago; 1974. University Press.
6. Polanyi M. *The Tacit Dimension.* Gloucester, MA: Peter Smith; 1983.
7. Charon, op cit.
8. Mishler EG. *The Discourse of Medicine: dialectics of medical interviews.* Norwood, NJ: Ablex Publishing Corp; 1984.
9. Said E. *Musical Elaborations.* London: Vintage; 1992.
10. Pelias R. Performative Writing as Scholarship: an apology, an argument, an anecdote. *Cultural Studies Critical Methodologies.* 2005; **54**: 415–24.
11. Ibid.
12. Becker G. *Disrupted Lives: how people create meaning in a chaotic world.* Berkeley and Los Angeles, CA: University of California Press; 1999.
13. Mattingly C. Performance narratives in the clinical world. In: Hurwitz B, Greenhalgh T, Skultans V, editors. *Narrative Research in Health and Illness.* Oxford: Blackwell Publishing; 2004.
14. Polkinghorne DE. Narrative configuration in qualitative analysis. In: Hatch JA, Wisniewski R, editors. *Life History and Narrative.* London: The Falmer Press; 1995.
15. Richardson L. *Writing Strategies: reaching diverse audiences.* Thousand Oaks, CA: Sage Qualitative Methodology Series; 1990.
16. Polkinghorne, op cit.
17. Etherington K. *Becoming a Reflexive Researcher: using our selves in research.* London: Jessica Kingsley; 2004.
18. Etherington K. *Trauma, the Body and Transformation.* London: Jessica Kingsley; 2003.
19. Etherington K. *Trauma, Drug Misuse and Transforming Identities.* London: Jessica Kingsley; 2008.
20. Polkinghorne, op cit.
21. Etherington, 2004, op cit.
22. Etherington, 2003, op cit.
23. Etherington, 2008, op cit.
24. Clough P. *Narratives and Fictions in Educational Research.* Buckingham: Open University Press; 2002.
25. Ellis C. *Final Negotiations.* Philadelphia, PA: Temple University Press; 1995.
26. Ellis C. Heartful ethnography. *Qualitative Health Research.* 1999; **9**(5): 669–83.
27. Ellis C. Creating criteria: an ethnographic short story. *Qualitative Inquiry.* 2000; **6**(2): 273–7.
28. Frank A. After Methods, the Story: from incongruity to truth. *Qualitative Research.* 2004a; **14**(3): 430–40.
29. Richardson, op cit.
30. Richardson L. The consequences of poetic representation: writing the other, rewriting the self. In: Ellis C, Flaherty M, editors. *Investigating Subjectivity: research on lived experience.* New York, NY: Sage; 1992.
31. Richardson L. Poetics, dramatics and transgressive validity: the case of the skipped line. In: *Sociol Q.* 1993; **34**(4): 695–710.

32. Richardson L. *Fields of Play (constructing an academic life)*. New Brunswick, NJ: Rutgers University Press; 1997.
33. Richardson L. Writing: a method of inquiry. In: Denzin NK, Lincoln YK, editors. *Handbook of Qualitative Research*. London: Sage; 2000.
34. Richardson L. Poetic representation of interviews. In: Gubrium J, Holstein JA, editors. *Handbook of Interview Research: context and method*. Thousand Oaks, CA: Sage; 2001b.
35. Sparkes A. *Telling Tales in Sport and Injury*. Champaign: Human Kinetics; 2002b.
36. Speedy J. *Narrative Inquiry and Psychotherapy*. Basingstoke: Palgrave Macmillan; 2008.
37. Frank A. *The Wounded Storyteller: body, illness and ethics*. Chicago, IL: University of Chicago Press; 1995.
38. Leach H. Crossing the line: stories on mapping the maze. *Times Higher Education Supplement*. 2004 Nov 5; pp. 18–19.
39. Bruner E. Ethnography as narrative. In: Turner V, Bruner E, editors. *The Anthropology of Experience*. Chicago, IL: University of Illinois Press; 1986.
40. Bird J. *The Heart's Narrative: therapy and navigating life's contradictions*. Auckland, New Zealand: Edge Press; 2000.
41. Martin V. *Out of my Head*. Lewes: Book Guild; 1997.
42. Martin V. A person centred perspective on the marginalising effects of illness and hospitalisation. *Auto/Biography*. 2000; 8(1 and 2): 19–26.
43. Martin V. Dialogue in the narrative process. *J Med Ethics*. 2007; 33: 49–54.
44. Capote T. *In Cold Blood*. London: The Reprint Society; 1967.
45. Thompson HS. *Fear and Loathing in Las Vegas*. New York, NY: Random House; 1971.
46. Wolfe T. *The New Journalism*. London: Picador; 1975.
47. Lodge D. The non-fiction novel. *The Independent on Sunday*. 1992 Apr 12.
48. Lodge D. The author's curse. *The Guardian*. 2006 May 20.
49. Wolfe, op cit.
50. Hunt C. *Therapeutic Dimensions of Autobiography in Creative Writing*. London: Jessica Kingsley; 2000.
51. Booth W. *The Rhetoric of Fiction*. Harmondsworth: Penguin; 1991.
52. Speedy, op cit.
53. Bruner, op cit.
54. Gee J. Units in the production of narrative discourse. *Discourse Processes*. 1986; 9: 391–422.
55. Gee J. A linguistic approach to narrative. *Journal of Narrative and Life History*. 1991; 1: 15–39.
56. McLeod J, Balamoutsou S. A method for qualitative narrative analysis for psychotherapy transcripts. In: Frommer J, Rennie DL, editors. *Qualitative Psychotherapy Research: Methods and Methodology*. Berlin: Pabst; 2000.
57. Richardson, 1990, op cit.
58. Richardson, 1992, op cit.
59. Richardson, 1993, op cit.
60. Richardson, 1997, op cit.
61. Richardson, 2000, op cit.
62. Richardson, 2001b, op cit.

63. Etherington, 2004, op cit.
64. Etherington, 2003, op cit.
65. Etherington, 2008, op cit.
66. Shotter J. Life inside dialogically structured mentalities: Bakhtin's and Voloshinov's account of our mental activities as out in the world between us. In: Rowan J, Cooper M, editors. *The Plural Self: multiplicity in everyday life.* London: Sage; 1999.
67. Richardson, 2001b, op cit.
68. Denzin N. *Interpretive Ethnography.* Thousand Oaks, CA: Sage; 1997.
69. Richardson, 2001b, op cit.
70. Richardson, 1990, op cit.
71. Richardson, 1992, op cit.
72. Richardson, 1993, op cit.
73. Richardson, 1997, op cit.
74. Richardson, 2000, op cit.
75. Richardson, 2001b, op cit.
76. Cixous H. *Three Steps on the Ladder of Writing.* New York, NY: Columbia University Press; 1993.
77. Martin, 2000, op cit.
78. Frank, op cit.
79. Williams R. *Marxism and Literature.* Oxford: Oxford University Press; 1977.
80. Rogers CR. *A Way of Being.* Boston, MA: Houghton Mifflin; 1980.
81. Clandinin J, Connelly FM. *Narrative Inquiry: experience and story in qualitative research.* San Francisco, CA: Jossey-Bass; 2000.
82. Pelias R. *A Methodology of the Heart: evoking academic and daily life.* Oxford: Alta Mira Press; 2004.
83. Ellis, 1999, op cit.
84. Sandelowski M. The proof of the pudding. In: Morse J, editor. *Critical Issues in Qualitative Research Methods.* London: Sage; 1994. pp. 46–63.
85. Charon, op cit.

CHAPTER 11

Implications and spaces

Oakley[1] ends her book *Fracture* with the hope that her quest for understanding the fracture of her right arm 'has uncovered commonalities in the human experience of embodiment and problems of health, illness and the body in our culture we need to address' (p. 154). I have a similar hope that my own quest for understanding, which I introduced in Chapter One, has illuminated the experience of illness, shed light on what constitutes helpful and healing practices, and indicated areas for further exploration and development.

The issues raised by the preceding stories, though situated, personal and particular, are relevant to all of us, whether patient, counsellor, researcher or healthcare professional. The narrators illustrate and give insight into what they needed as patients from healthcare professionals and carers. In doing so, they contribute narrative knowledge which can enhance the practice of ethical and 'aesthetic medicine'.[2] By focusing on the singularity of each of the storytellers, offering personal understandings, intentions and meanings, I have hoped to inform and move the reader, and to challenge the polarised positioning of patient and practitioner, client and counsellor, researcher and researched. We will all be patients at some point in our lives; illness and mortality are not what happen to others, but are a condition of being embodied human beings subject to contingency. As Charon[3] expresses it, intersubjective approaches to healthcare ethics 'seek congress among human beings limited by mortality, identified by culture, revealed in language, and marked by suffering. It is not the case that some are sick and some are well but that all will die' (p. 27).

As I draw together the threads of understanding from the five stories on which this book has focused, I aim to highlight ways in which the issues that they raise may contribute to healthcare research and practice. In the concluding chapter of *Trauma, the Body and Transformation*, Etherington[4] writes:

> I see myself as a weaver, a tapestry maker, whose tale is created from the threads that arise from the stories which have gone before … The threads that I weave into this chapter may be different from those that you have used, because you and I bring different things to the reading: our histories, our perceptions, our prior knowledge. (p. 180)

I believe the concerns raised by the storytellers have implications for healthcare, and for future research. However, like Etherington, I recognise that each reader will approach these stories from a different frame of reference, and therefore weave her/his own threads of experience into the tapestry of this book.

In relation to the notion of embodiment and issues of de-personalisation, I will focus on the importance of relationships between healthcare professionals and patients. With regard to issues of limbo, I will consider issues such as continuity of care, which involves healthcare policy and making provision to support staff in their efforts to deliver humane and effective healthcare.

WHAT DOES IT MEAN TO BE TREATED 'AS A PERSON'?

Relationships between healthcare professionals and patients clearly play an important role in healthcare settings. As each of the storytellers has indicated, the need to be related to 'as a person' is of prime importance when we are positioned as patients. I want to examine here what this actually means in practice, before going on to consider ways in which this might be fostered.

In my view, fundamental dimensions of 'relating as a person' are those qualities that Carl Rogers[5,6] referred to as the 'core conditions': empathy, congruence and unconditional positive regard. Their place in counselling and psychotherapy has long been recognised, though given different emphasis according to theoretical orientation. I will focus particularly on empathy in this discussion, since it has also gained some attention in the literature relating to healthcare practice, notably in the work of Spiro *et al.*,[7] and Charon,[8,9,10] who links the capacity for empathy with the development of 'narrative competence'. I regard empathy as one of the key means of reaching across the divide between the ill and those who care for the ill. The isolation of illness to which each of the stories testifies can therefore be, if not diminished to some degree, then acknowledged by the willingness to engage in the suffering of the other. Charon[11] draws on Levinas' concepts of the 'face' and of responsibility to be open to the call of another who suffers. She writes, 'When we are called forth in the Levinasian sense, by the other's face in a clinical setting, we are called forth to join patients in the fear and pain of illness or nearness to death' (p. 135).

Empathy, according to Rogers,[12] is a process of 'entering the private perceptual world of the other' (p. 142), and of sensing, as closely as possible, the subjective experiencing of another person. It involves being open to personal resonance, but has an 'as if' quality that distinguishes it from identification, and therefore it fundamentally requires a sensitivity to and awareness of *difference*: we can never fully enter into the consciousness of another human being, or fully experience the world as another experiences it. Nevertheless, I believe that the willingness to engage with the suffering of another and to offer one's presence is an important dimension of humane healthcare. As Charon[13] writes of narrative approaches to medicine, 'One wants to join with the patient, as a whole presence, deploying all one's human gifts of intuition, empathy and ability to bear witness to each patient one sees' (p. 133).

Davies'[14] describes empathy as a 'warm fuzzy pursuit' (p. 19), and indeed it is often characterised (or perhaps, caricatured) as such. However, in my view, it is a quality that requires considerable risk on the part of both storyteller and listener. As a story-*teller*, one can find empathy quite daunting: to be understood in all one's complexity and ambiguity can be deeply challenging. When we are offered the sensitivity and subtlety of full empathic engagement, which touches the 'edge of awareness' and enables the possibility of exploring subjective experience, we venture into uncertain territory.[15] As empathic story-*listeners* we draw on our full emotional, affective, intuitive, cognitive and linguistic capacities in order to offer empathic companionship to another. Such empathic engagement is demanding, and involves deep and close attention—alongside respect—for the storyteller; it involves tentatively communicating and checking our understanding, and awareness of potential 'blocks to communication'[16] (p. 92) that can impede empathic listening.

I will reflect a little on my own empathic process here because I think it has some bearing on empathy within the patient/healthcare professional relationship. As a counsellor, my experience is that when I can move fully and delicately through and with the experiencing of another person at the same time as being firmly connected to the source and ground of my own being, this can be a reciprocal and healing feature of the therapeutic relationship. I think empathy requires imagination, delicacy and compassion as well as intuition, sensitivity and attunement to what Mearns and Thorne[17] term the 'personal language' (p. 64) of another. An openness to one's own resonance is, in my view, a fundamental dimension of the empathic process, and can act as a personal reference point that we can choose to access in order to 'release empathic sensitivity'[18] (p. 53). In working with the storytellers, it was important for me, in conjunction with my principal research supervisor, to monitor dynamics of projection, identification, projective identification and counter-transference. I think there were times when my empathy blurred with identification, but I also came to realise that my personal resonance and recognition informed my empathy and opened up areas for stories that may not have been told. This was important in subverting the power dynamics of researcher and researched. (At the same time, I feel that my decision *not* to seek a participant with brain injury was the right decision for me. I felt the possibility of my over-identification was more likely, and that this would have impeded the process of empathic engagement with the uniqueness and difference of another's experience.)

In my relationships with participants, I needed to remain aware of the potential for the mechanisms of projective identification and counter-transference, in which my emotional response to the storytellers could involve my taking on the feelings of each contributor as if they were my own. Conversely, I needed to acknowledge the potential for my own defence mechanisms, in which I might project my fears onto the contributors.

Tansey and Burke[19] argue that projective identification is an important dimension of the empathic process. Peter Martin[20] (p. 239–30) also regards this as integral to empathy and writes, 'Work at the edge seems to involve the pain of recognition' and 'the flash of identity'. He adds, 'I would tend to *privilege* the stage of identification, as being necessary to be a witness', while at the same time recognising 'that continuous identification is not the same as empathy', but rather a 'process of drawing towards and drawing away allowed for moments of identification which were then held in tension by withdrawal and reflection'. As a counsellor, and as a researcher, my experience is that the process of empathic engagement involves moments of recognition as well as reflection and further exploration.

Empathy has certainly been recognised as playing an important role in the relationships between patient and healthcare practitioners. Larsen and Xin Yao[21] argue that making connections and 'developing empathy are fundamental to caring and enhance the therapeutic potential of patient-clinician relationships' (p. 1100). Stepien and Baernstein[22] report that 'empathy is believed to significantly influence patient satisfaction, adherence to medical recommendations, clinical outcomes, and professional satisfaction' (p. 524).

Linked to empathy is the capacity to be fully present; like empathy, 'presence' is a difficult concept to define or to pin down. It can have an almost transcendental quality; as Rogers[23] writes: 'it seems that my inner spirit has reached out and touched the inner spirit of the other' (p. 129). But equally it can be the capacity not to turn away, such as that demonstrated by Yasmin's doctor. Charon[24] writes of 'taking care of a gravely ill elderly man' when she 'was an intern—sleep-deprived, unused to my authority, unsure of what to do for this patient' who was 'irretrievably sick', and of how while she knew how to manage his physical needs, she did not know how 'to manage the fact of his dying', 'his wife's fear and loss' nor 'my own suffering in the face of theirs'. She notes, 'I did not know that I was allowed as a doctor to donate my presence, my attention, my regard', and demonstrates her incipient recognition of the healing potential of such genuine, respectful 'presence' (p. 34).

However, as Wilson and Lindy[25] point out, professionals such as healthcare practitioners and social workers who work with trauma 'not only confront the pain and personal struggle of the client but must do so with a capacity for sustained empathy'; this can leave them vulnerable to 'empathic strain ... making it difficult to stay closely attuned ...' (p. 1).

HOW CAN 'RELATING AS A PERSON' WITH THE CAPACITY FOR EMPATHY AND PRESENCE BE FOSTERED AND SUPPORTED?

If we regard empathy as an important quality of relationships in healthcare, this raises questions of how it might be fostered, and also of how healthcare professionals can be supported in managing empathic strain. Within the field of therapy, practitioners have ongoing supervision, where issues such as counter-transference and projective identification can be addressed. However, many healthcare professionals who are faced daily with the trauma associated with illness do not have access to such a system of 'supervision'. As Wilson and Lindy[26] note:

> Successful management of empathic strain facilitates the maintenance of an empathic stance. To suggest that this very human process is easily accomplished would be misleading; at the very least it demands that therapists be open to their own feelings and experiences and that they rely on collegial consultation and supervision. (p. 34)

Therefore it would seem to be in the interests of healthcare professionals as well as patients that there is access to safe space, time and opportunity for reflection on personal and professional issues.

Charon[27] has developed an approach to practice that she terms 'Narrative Medicine': this signifies 'a clinical practice informed by the theory and practice of reading, writing, telling and rereading of stories' and was motivated by her sense that 'what medicine *lacks* today—in singularity, humility, accountability, empathy—can in part be provided through intensive narrative training' (p. viii). One of the primary ways by which Charon[28] enables the development of the qualities of narrative competence is through a device for reflective writing known as the 'Parallel Chart' (p. 155), by which students reflect on their personal responses to patients. This is not a general piece of reflective writing such as a journal, but rather 'narrative writing in the service of the care of a particular patient' (p. 157). The students then read this writing to their fellow students once a week in a session devoted specifically to sharing and developing awareness and personal learning. The aim of this writing is primarily to enable students 'to recognize more fully what their patients endure and to examine explicitly their own journeys through medicine.' Charon regards it as an 'essential part of medical training, designed to increase the students' capacity for effective clinical work', which students have found beneficial:

> Writers found they understood their own emotions more clearly by virtue of writing and reading aloud of their experience. They also found that they understood their patients more fully. (p. 173)

She reports that ongoing research into the outcomes of this writing showed that students were 'more effective in conducting medical interviews, performing medical procedures, and developing therapeutic alliances with patients' (p. 174).

Pennebaker[29] found that narrative writing in relation to personal trauma, integrated thought and feeling, brought meaning and structure to experience and 'seemed to be critical in reaching understanding' (p. 10). It also reduced isolation by enabling 'a richer connection between the storytellers and their social networks' (p. 14). Reflective writing and witnessing such as that described by Charon could similarly bring about a sense of connection and mutual support within the 'social network' of healthcare staff. Writing as a process of exploration can lead to greater awareness, understanding and discovery. It can help to develop awareness of professional as well as personal issues, enhance critical thinking, and enable the consideration of issues such as language, knowledge and power. Bolton[30] demonstrates how the engagement in such reflective practice can lead to the development of greater insight, sensitivity and critical examination of professional practice.

Such an approach to reflective writing has been successfully used with final-year medical students at the University of Bristol Medical School during a course in which they 'shadow' doctors in the post that they will go on to take up following graduation. Their reflections highlight not only the formative process of their learning, but also offer insight into what is required within medical education. Sir Kenneth Calman, in his foreword to the collection of their accounts edited by Feest and Forbes[31] (p. v), described the book as 'inspirational and should be read by all who have any part to play in the education of doctors'. The book shows how the opportunity for reflective writing can highlight the collective nature of healthcare and contribute to better understanding. As Feest and Forbes (p. x) note of the students, 'Their observations will help both service providers and patients to more fully understand some of the tensions that are inherent within the present healthcare system'.

Jan's comments on the culture of the ward round, where personal interaction is hierarchical between e.g. consultant and medical student, show how such values can impact on the patient, who becomes the focus or object of such a teaching method. Alternative approaches to ward round learning are suggested by Bleakley *et al.*,[32] who take account of the 'hidden curriculum'[33] of medical education and advocate models of learning that are not based solely on the transmission of knowledge and skills. They challenge the polarisation of science and the arts/humanities and propose a view of the medical curriculum as 'an aesthetic text and learning as aesthetic and ethical identity formation' (p. 197). Thus, learning is seen as a forming and formative process that takes account of the socialisation within communities of practice. By drawing on concepts as diverse as the poststructural thinking of Foucault[34] and Deleuze[35] and Polanyi's[36] notion of 'indwelling', they offer an aesthetic and integrated approach to medical humanities as 'process and perspective rather than content … with a function not only to support learning of knowledge and skills but also learning of values and attributes that constitute an identity' (p. 197). Thus a humanities-based ward round might include attention to stories, to rhetorical strategies, to acts of witnessing and empathy which deepen 'the perceptual capabilities and moral imagination of student' (p. 210). Such an approach therefore includes the patient as a member of a collaborative learning community rather than a depersonalised focus of teaching.

Marshall and Kelley's[37] (p. 114) description of a poetry workshop for healthcare staff illustrates how the capacity for 'relating as a person' is fostered through the aesthetic *tending* and telling of one's own stories and *attending to* one another's stories. They write:

> Participants realised that another was voicing their problems; that there was a real sharing of which they had been unaware; above all that there were real talents among their peers for giving a new voice to common and sometimes old problems.

The poems included in their article are deeply moving and tackle serious issues with poignant and piercing beauty (p. 115–116). As Feest and Forbes[38] demonstrate in their collection of students' accounts, when medical education includes opportunities for reflective writing, it gives students 'permission' to be vulnerable, and in that expression, permission to be open and attuned to the stories, vulnerabilities and strengths of their patients. I believe it is through such reflexive and reflective practices that the stories of healthcare professionals and those of patients can reach across the divisions between the sick and the well, and enhance the learning of all concerned.

I recall an occasion in hospital when two medical students came to talk to me; it was shortly before my consultant's ward round, and they had come to familiarise themselves with my 'case'. They were very sweet, gentle, respectful, curious and keen to 'learn' from the patient. Their genuine interest and willingness to engage with me in a collaborative learning process—in which we learnt from each other—was affirming for me as a patient and also paid dividends when they 'impressed' my consultant with their understanding. It was an example of the way education does not need to be hierarchical to be effective. Medical education can be more collective and inclusive; it can and should include medical students, staff and patients as members of a community of practice in which learning is drawn from experience and collaboration as well as a scientific, medical knowledge base.

The 'shadowing' scheme described by Feest and Forbes[39] reminds us that as practitioners, counsellors, patients, we are all human beings—embodied, vulnerable and mortal. Telling our stories and attending the stories of others is a responsibility to others and to ourselves.

TIME AND CONTINUITY OF CARE

When I asked Yasmin what message she particularly wanted to convey to medical practitioners, she replied, 'I think that doctors these days are far too busy; there's too much pressure on them. And there are far too many things demanding their attention all the time. And the patients suffer. Like when I go to out-patients to see my doctor I always feel pressured and I can't go in and sit down and say to him this is what I'm like because there are people waiting outside and he's already half an hour late.' As Bleakley *et al.*,[40] (p. 205) note, 'doctors are increasingly compromised in their work by rapidly changing institutional frameworks such as health service targets and health care bureaucracy, which invite dissimulation.'

Yasmin was frequently admitted to hospital as an emergency. An on-call doctor late at night would not have access to her very detailed notes. The onus was on Yasmin or her companion to briefly explain the complexity of her condition. A personal record card, which summarises the details of a condition such as Yasmin's and which can be kept by the patient and taken in, would be helpful. In a practice comparable to the use of documents in narrative therapy,[41] Charon[42] has 'come slowly to appreciate that patients should be the curators of what we write about them. At the conclusion of visits, I give patients a copy of my chart note … encouraging them to add to what has been said on the next visit' (p. 190).

Pharmacist Koda-Kimble,[43] tells the moving story of her sister, who suffered from bowel cancer for 14 years, and asks, 'How can we as educators provide our students with experiences that help them begin to see how care looks and feels from the patient's and family's perspective?' (p. 5) She makes a wide range of practical, professionally informed, compassionate suggestions, which include encouraging students to evaluate existing systems and practices in relation to continuity of care, and to think actively about ways of enhancing patient care. In addition, she makes the following suggestion, which involves providing students with 'at least one experience that allows the student to travel the health care road alongside the patient'. This might involve 'sitting at a patient's bedside for 24 to 48 hours, as would a close member of the family, or working with a patient from home to clinic to pharmacy to home again'. She observes that these 'kinds of experiences would allow the student to observe the ebb and flow of care; comprehend the jagged nature of a patient's health status; get a sense of the worry, fear, sadness, and impatience the patient and their families experience as they navigate the health care system when they are most vulnerable' (p. 5).

Perhaps healthcare professionals who have experienced serious illness, or those such as Koda-Kimble who have experienced a close family member or friend being ill, are in a position to know what is needed but also what is possible within the constraints of a system where increasing demands are being made on staff. I believe their stories would further illuminate healthcare practice and offer powerful lessons not just about what we require in illness and why, but about how those needs can be most humanely served by practitioners within a hospital setting—and that this might be an area with potential for future research.

PRACTICES WITHIN MEDICAL EDUCATION AND CONTINUING PROFESSIONAL DEVELOPMENT THAT THIS RESEARCH SUPPORTS

Narrative approaches position people alongside each other and therefore recognise the reciprocal nature of conversations between storytellers and audience.[44]

I do not presume to make recommendations for practice but rather offer the following as practices that this study supports. This research is partial, contingent and in line with narrative ethics and the relational and collaborative position I have taken throughout; it is offered by my participants and by me as an invitation to a prospective audience, whether student or qualified practitioner. Practices that are supported by this research might include:

- Exercises to foster practitioners' awareness of their own personal embodiment.
- Exercises that will sensitise practitioners to issues such as isolation, limbo, depersonalisation/mortality.
- Opportunities to develop critical awareness of language and discourse.
- Exercises to develop awareness of imagery; if we listen for metaphoric language in ourselves and in others, we can become more aware of the meanings and power of socially sanctioned analogies, and challenge those that are unhelpful.
- Opportunities to develop creative, playful, imaginative use of figurative language through poetry, outsider witness practices and writing fiction.
- Activities such as those used in counselling training to develop critical awareness of active listening processes and skill.[45]

ADDITIONAL NARRATIVE PRACTICES MIGHT INCLUDE:

- The writing of 'Parallel Charts',[46] in which practitioners write personal responses in relation to a particular patient as part of mainstream, continuing professional development.
- The reading aloud and discussion of 'Parallel Charts' as part of continuing personal and professional development.
- Narrative reflective practice: a way of using 'Parallel Charts' that uses Clandinin and Connelly's three-dimensional narrative inquiry practices;[47] using the group process for exploring 'Parallel Charts' along dimensions of temporality, personal/social context and context of place or landscape. Clandinin and Cave[48] develop Charon's idea of the 'Parallel Chart' as a means of narrative reflective practice and note the beneficial impact on clinical skills: 'It's not just about feeling good, or helping patients feel good. It actually makes a difference to diagnosis and management. It's actually clinically relevant, honing those skills, the stuff we don't have time to think about which is meaningful for that particular patient'.[49]
- Telling and re-telling of stories in the context of outsider witness practices and reflecting teams.[50,51]
- Opportunities to read/discuss/write practitioner stories as a means of creating peer support.

WRITING OPPORTUNITIES MIGHT INCLUDE:

- Creating a literature/reading group for discussions and also as a context/ stimulus for creative writing practices.
- Writing patients' stories from the perspective of that patient.
- Opportunities for writing such as Feest and Forbes[52] collection of medical students' writing.
- Writing practices such as those in 'The Gift', which celebrates the work of healthcare practitioners and where the contributors include not only established writers such as Doris Lessing and Hanif Kureishi, but also the staff in the NHS in Birmingham, and in which 'the writers hope that their work might inspire medical workers to reflect on how people who use their service feel and think about their experience'.[53]

REFLECTIVE PRACTICES MIGHT INCLUDE:

- Challenges to reflect on the dominant cultural forces and to enable questioning and examination of ideology and discourses in medicine.
- Explicit exploration of aspects of the 'hidden curriculum'.
- Opportunities to evaluate and think critically about existing systems and practices.
- Opportunities for practitioners to think how they might modify their own practices in ways that enhance patient experiences.
- Challenges to students to think actively and imaginatively about how, if they were in charge, things might be done differently in situations that are not ideal.

MEDICAL PRACTICES AND POLICIES MIGHT INCLUDE:

- The opportunity for consultations where the emphasis is on 'how is this affecting your life?' as a matter of course.
- A system of 'supervision' for staff such as that used in counselling and psychotherapy which promotes and encourages self-awareness and reflexive practice alongside critical reflection.
- Training and support in counselling skill relevant and appropriate to a relational narrative approach to medicine including the exploration of meanings of person/patient-centred.

REFERENCES

1. Oakley A. *Fracture: adventures of a broken body.* Bristol: The Policy Press; 2007.
2. Bleakley A, Marshall R, Bromer R. Toward an aesthetic medicine: developing a core medical humanities undergraduate curriculum. *J Med Human.* 2006; **27**: 197–213.

3. Charon R. The ethicality of narrative medicine. In: Hurwitz B, Greenhalgh T, Skultans V, editors. *Narrative Research in Health and Illness.* London: BMJ Books; 2004.

4. Etherington K. *Trauma, the Body and Transformation.* London: Jessica Kingsley; 2003.

5. Rogers CR. *On Becoming a Person.* Boston, MA: Houghton Mifflin; 1961.

6. Rogers CR. *A Way of Being.* Boston: Houghton Mifflin; 1980.

7. Spiro HM, McCrea C, Curnen MG, *et al.*, editors. *Empathy and the Practice of Medicine.* London: Yale University Press; 1993.

8. Charon R. *Narrative Medicine: honoring the stories of illness.* Oxford: Oxford University Press; 2006.

9. Charon R. The narrative road to empathy. In: Spiro HM, McCrea C, Curnen MG, *et al.*, editors. *Empathy and the Practice of Medicine: beyond pills and the scalpel.* London: Yale University Press; 1993.

10. Charon R. Narrative medicine: a model for empathy, reflection, profession and trust. *JAMA.* 2001; **286**(15): 1897–902.

11. Charon, 2006, op cit.

12. Rogers, 1961, op cit.

13. Charon, 2006, op cit.

14. Davies B. *A body of writing, 1989–1999.* Walnut Creek, CA: Alta Mira Press; 2000.

15. Gendlin E. The client's client: the edge of awareness. In: Levant R, Schlien J, editors. *Client-Centered Therapy and the Person-Centered Approach: new directions in theory, research and practice.* New York, NY: Praeger; 1984. pp. 76–110.

16. Merry T. *Learning and Being in Person-Centred Counselling.* Ross-on-Wye: PCCS Books; 1999.

17. Mearns D, Thorne B. *Person-Centred Counselling in Action.* London: Sage; 1988.

18. Ibid.

19. Tansey MJ, Burke WF. *Understanding Countertransference: from projective identification to empathy.* Taylor & Francis; 1989.

20. Martin P. *The Effect of Personal Life Events on the Practice of Therapists* [unpublished PhD thesis]. 2005.

21. Larsen E, Yao X. Clinical empathy as emotional labor in the patient-physician relationship. *JAMA.* 2005; **293**(9): 1100–6.

22. Stepien K, Baernstein A. Educating for empathy. *J Gen Intern Med.* 2006; **21**: 524–30.

23. Rogers, 1961, op cit.

24. Charon, 2006, op cit.

25. Wilson JP, Lindy JD. *Countertransference in the Treatment of PTSD.* New York, NY: Guilford Press; 1994.

26. Ibid.

27. Charon, 2006, op cit.

28. Charon, 2006, op cit.

29. Pennebaker JW. Telling stories: the health benefits of narrative. *Lit Med.* 2000; **19**(1): 3–18.

30. Bolton G. *Reflective Practice: writing and professional development.* 2005; London: Sage.

31. Feest K, Forbes K. *Today's Students, Tomorrow's Doctors.* Oxford: Radcliffe; 2007.

32. Bleakley, Marshall, Bromer, op cit.

33. Jackson P. Life in classrooms. 1968. In: Pollard B, Bourne J. *Teaching and Learning in the Primary School.* London: Routledge; 1994.

34. Foucault M. *Power/Knowledge: selected interviews and other writings.* Gordon C, editor. New York, NY: Pantheon Books; 1980.
35. Deleuze G, Guattari F. *A thousand plateaus.* London: Athlone Press; 1987.
36. Polanyi M, Prosch H. *Meaning.* Chicago, IL: The University of Chicago Press; 1977.
37. Marshall R, Kelley A. Opening the word hoard. *J Med Ethics.* 2006; **32**: 114–16.
38. Feest, Forbes, op cit.
39. Ibid.
40. Bleakley, Marshall, Bromer, op cit.
41. White M, Epston D. *Narrative Means to Therapeutic Ends.* New York, NY: Norton; 1990.
42. Charon, 2006, op cit.
43. Koda-Kimble M. A patient's "tail": lessons from the bedside. *Am J Pharm Educ.* 2004; **68**(3); Article 70.
44. Speedy J. *Narrative Inquiry and Psychotherapy.* Basingstoke: Palgrave Macmillan; 2008.
45. McLeod J. *Narrative and Psychotherapy.* London: Sage; 1997.
46. Charon, 2006, op cit.
47. Clandinin J, Connelly FM. *Narrative Inquiry: experience and story in qualitative research.* San Francisco, CA: Jossey-Bass; 2000.
48. Clandinin J, Cave M. Creating pedagogical spaces for developing doctor professional identity. *Med Educ.* 2008; **42**: 765–70.
49. Clandinin J, Cave M. Storytelling in medicine. Available at: www.expressnews.ualberta.ca/article.cfm?id=8246.
50. White M, Epston D. *Narrative Means to Therapeutic Ends.* New York, NY: Norton; 1990.
51. White M. Reflecting teamwork as definitional ceremony re-visited. In *Gecko: A journal of deconstruction and narrative ideas in therapeutic practice.* Adelaide: Dulwich Centre Publications; 1999.
52. Feest, Forbes, op cit.
53. Morley D, editor. *The Gift: new writing for the NHS.* Exeter: Stride Publications (in association with Birmingham Health Authority); 2002.

CHAPTER 12

Evolution and reflection

In this chapter I reflect on the evolution of my particular approach to narrative inquiry. After offering a critique of the person-centred approach as a research methodology, I will conclude the chapter and draw this book to a close by returning briefly to the autoethnographic voice I used in Chapter One.

FROM COUNSELLOR TO RESEARCHER: SOME METHODOLOGICAL REFLECTIONS

As a counsellor, I have listened to stories unfold and worked in collaboration with clients to explore experience, events and meanings. When I ventured into research, I was relatively confident that I had the qualities and professional skills to participate in the telling of stories of serious illness and its impact on people's lives, but knew that I had much to learn. I was aware that the purposes of therapy and research were different, and that rather than being in a 'helping' role, I was undertaking a research project where participants would be helping *me* to develop and explore my ideas and understandings of illness against the social and cultural backdrop of early 21st century England in order to illuminate and contribute to healthcare practice and policy. Unlike many counsellors who move into research, I was not researching counselling *per se*: I was neither investigating the counselling process nor its outcomes. Rather I was interested in the complexity and uniqueness of illness experience within the context of a life, and how this influenced and affected people's sense of self and identity. I wanted to investigate the stories people told of illness, to develop a means of representing them in such a way as to touch the hearts and minds of listeners and readers, and thus to contribute to the mosaic of knowledge within the field of healthcare.

I was aware that undertaking research would require the development of additional skills and knowledge, and I certainly found that the transition from counsellor to researcher presented me with challenges. My early research conversations with Pat and with Jan were a particularly important part of my learning, and when I started working with Pat, I was still strongly in 'counsellor mode', and far *more* so than I had initially realised. I came to recognise that the way I was engaging with Pat was limiting both the range of stories Pat could tell, and also the way in which such stories could be told. While I could see that I was sufficiently empathic, accepting and genuine in the relationship to enable Pat to explore her experience in some depth, what I did *not* see was the way in which this mode of relating kept her focus *inward*. Pat later told me that she had found the first session helpful in a cathartic way, but that it had felt more to her like counselling than research. While I clearly consider empathy to be very important in research, my empathic 'tracking', reflection and paraphrasing, which in a counselling relationship can facilitate the expression and exploration of experience, seemed to limit the range of stories rather than open out to new possibilities of multiple stories.

My learning in relation to eliciting 'data' fell broadly into two main areas: my use of focused questions, and my use of personal resonance. In my first meetings with Pat and Jan, I tended to linger within the 'landscape of consciousness'.[1] This had the effect at times of restricting conversations to the terrain of meanings and values, whereas the more direct questioning stance I later used focused equally on events, on sequence, on eliciting details of particular incidents, on embodied sensory details, as well as on details of social setting and context. I found that 'scaffolding' more effectively between 'landscapes' enabled a richer storying of events as well as exploration of thoughts, meaning and feelings. I am also very aware that I have much to learn, to develop my skills and qualities as a narrative researcher.

In the table below, I offer a summary of the limitations of the person-centred approach as a means of research, and follow this with a summary of the salient advantages offered by postmodern approaches to narrative research.

Summary of the limitations of the person–centred approach to research

The person-centred approach requires rigorous training, experience and practice; while often characterised (and at times caricatured) as soft, gentle and non-directive, it requires discipline, self-monitoring and critical reflection. The translation of the core conditions of empathy, unconditional regard and congruence into therapeutic skills demands self-awareness, focused and intensive personal development work, as well as rigorous consultation through the supervision process. Empathy may be equated and confused with identification. For example, Spiro[2] (p. 2) introduces a collection of essays with the following: 'Empathy is the feeling that "I might be you" or "I am you" but it is more than just an intellectual identification; empathy must be accompanied by feeling'. This common oversimplification of the empathic *process* fails to take account of the place of *difference* in empathy. It is *not* how 'I might feel in your situation' but rather a delicate and subtle sensing of the frame of reference of the other person, an awareness by the counsellor of his/her own points of reference, and decisions made in the moment of whether and how to use personal resonance. Empathy requires, in Levinas'[3] terms, recognition of the extent to which we can never ultimately know another person's subjective experience. The feasibility of using empathy in research conversations therefore requires skill and experience, as well as recognition of the affective load of working at 'relational depth'.

Such an in-depth approach to narrative research requires understanding of the role of one's own stories and personal needs, such that a researcher can *choose* to access and use personal resonance when appropriate and facilitative.

The person-centred approach *on its own* can tend to keep the participant's focus inwards. While working in a person-centred way can facilitate experiential processing and exploration of meanings, it is less effective at eliciting details of social context, the place of other characters, temporal accounts of events, causality and plot.

This approach can tend to dwell in the landscape of consciousness: on experiential processing, and reflection on meanings.

Narrative approaches to research, on the other hand, can elicit stories[4] since they take into account the following:

Salient features of narrative approaches to research

- Events
- Temporality and sequencing, as well as messiness and disorder
- Intentionality and agency: choices, actions and reasons
- Causality, plot and meaning
- Other characters
- Personal embodied detail: senses, feelings, thoughts, ideas, sensory details—sights, sounds, smells
- Details that evoke cultural and social context
- The 'absent but implicit', which allows the acknowledgement of paradox, contradiction and ambiguity[5]
- The thickening and enriching of habitually told stories
- The ways people create and construct identity and meaning
- The potential for examining taken-for-granted storylines, received notions and social myths

I suggest that a combination of the qualities of the person-centred approach with the questioning stance of narrative inquiry allows for effective scaffolding between landscapes of action and consciousness. A relational way of working takes account of the dialogic in the narrative process. Both the person-centred approach and the narrative approach of those such as White and Epston,[6] Etherington,[7,8,9,10,11] Payne,[12] and Speedy[13,14] start from a 'not knowing' stance,[15] where the therapist or researcher refuses to adopt the role of expert, and where the professionalised 'language of deficit', as described by Gergen[16] and associated with other therapeutic approaches, is challenged.

DIALOGUE: A RELATIONAL NARRATIVE APPROACH

An important stage of my learning was in my writing and reflection, which led to conference presentations on this relational narrative approach and a subsequent article, 'Dialogue in the Narrative Process'.[17] In these writings I focused on Pat's story and set out to capture a sense of the relational nature of our research conversations, to convey the many dimensions of engaging in a dialogic way, and also to explore the conceptual aspects of 'dialogue' from the perspectives of Martin Buber and Mikhail Bakhtin, and with regard to certain sites of dialogue: within the research relationship; within the research process; within the individual; and between the text and the reader. I draw on that article in the following reflections.

DIALOGUE AND HETEROTOPIC SPACE[18]

My counselling training had emphasised 'bracketing' in the sense derived from Husserl's phenomenology; this view of reality as perceived and as subjectively experienced regards therapeutic change as associated with understanding another person's worldview or 'frame of reference' as fully and empathically as possible. As a counsellor, I tried to be as aware as possible of the ways in which my own 'frame of reference' could obscure a clear appreciation of another person's subjective reality, and then to 'bracket' this off. I was very disciplined and cautious about disclosing my own experience, neither wanting to make assumptions about another person's frame of reference nor to shift attention from client to counsellor. However, during the early meetings with Pat, and also with Jan, I became aware that I was 'bracketing' in a way that was unhelpful and was not dialogic in Buber's[19] sense of *I-Thou* relating, but was effectively keeping me 'safe', as well as inhibiting an exploration of areas of shared experience. However, as Rogers[20] (p. 27) points out:

> The very feeling which has seemed to me most private, most personal, and hence most incomprehensible by others, has turned out to be an expression for which there is a resonance in many other people.

As a counsellor, I would ask myself whether self-disclosure would move the therapeutic process on, and I would err on the side of caution. I came to realise that in research an expression of personal resonance could open up further areas for exploration and co-construction; by expressing, for example, my own sense of mortality, this created a space for Pat to talk about her thoughts and feelings relating to death. Thus, in tentatively offering my own experience, I was offering a kind of 'heterotopic space'[21] (a concept developed by Foucault to refer to spaces that have dual meanings) where others might see reflection as well as difference. And this has not been a matter of simple expediency, but one concerning whether I could carry out my research aims with integrity and with respect for the integrity of the other person. Was I willing and able to relate as a person, to 'be' in relation? And was this possible within a research relationship?

Buber[22] accepts that both *I-Thou* and *I-It* modes of relating are necessary; he states, 'Without *It* a man cannot live. But he who lives with *It* alone is not a man' (p. 52). Clearly in research there is a purpose, an objective, so arguably there is an objectification of the person, and thus an *I-It* dimension; but I would still contend that there can be fleeting *I-Thou* moments in which there is a shift from 'communication to communion'[23] (p. 6), and which can therefore be transforming for both researcher and participant. As Rogers[24] writes: 'Such a deep and mutual personal encounter doesn't happen often, but I am convinced that unless it happens occasionally, we are not living fully as human beings' (p. 19). I think that where there is a commitment to relating equally, in a dialogic way, and a willingness to engage fully, then there is no reason why we cannot be open to such moments in the research relationship. Indeed, Frank[25] contends that a dialogical approach to research is both empirical, in the sense that research relationships are 'interactive and reactive', and also 'ethically desirable' (p. 973).

DIALOGUE WITHIN THE RESEARCH PROCESS

There is a dialogic and dynamic element within the research process itself where our conversations can impact on that which is being researched, and also on each person's sense of self, in a way that is dynamic and transformative. Frank[26] writes, 'The struggle for most ill people seems to be keeping multiple selves available to themselves' (p. 66). As Frank suggests, telling stories is, perhaps, one of the ways in which those selves can be created.

I learnt a great deal from asking Pat and Jan what was helpful to them in the research process; and this influenced my sense of self as a researcher, such as in the development of my confidence and sensitivity in knowing when or how to disclose aspects of my own experience. For example, when I asked Pat about the occasions when I had referred to my own illness, she said, 'I feel it was important as it showed you were involved; otherwise you would have had all the power and the relationship would have been unequal and uneven', and felt that this was something I should disclose with other participants. Jan had similarly found it helpful and had told me that where there was resonance it 'helped the flow of the conversation' and acted as 'a kind of reflection and a summary of what I've been saying or a chance to think about it in a slightly different way', thus perhaps indicating a sense of 'hetero-topia' as a type of mirror and 'site of alternate ordering'[27] (p. 24). Therefore, when I met Jim and Yasmin, I was more aware and also more experienced in offering that kind of reciprocity.

DIALOGUE WITHIN THE INDIVIDUAL: AMBIGUITY AND INTERSUBJECTIVITY

Another element of dialogue is that within each individual—the 'internal dia-logue' between different aspects of ourselves, as well as the dialogues we each carry between others present or absent (partners, children, medical people and so on). Bakhtin suggests that such dialogue both informs and is informed by things that have been said before; language does not operate in a vacuum but is dynamic and intersubjective. In *The Problems of Dostoevsky's Poetics*,[28] he describes Dostoevsky's predisposition to dialogism as follows:

> In every voice he could hear two contending voices, in every expression a crack, and the readiness to go over immediately to another contradictory expression; in every gesture he detected confidence and lack of confidence simultaneously; he perceived the profound ambiguity, even multiple ambiguity, of every phenom-enon. (p. 30)

My understanding of Bakhtin's reference to 'voices' is of the multiplicity of voices within each of us and within the text—the complexity, contradiction and ambigu-ity of those voices, as well as the way our language is infused with the voices of others. For example, we hear Pat preparing herself for the possibility of dying: 'I'd made my peace', followed by the angry self who feels 'cheated' when she wakes up and finds that she is alive, the rebel who challenges the orthodoxy of 'I'm lucky to be alive' and subverts the passivity of patienthood. We hear the mischievous, playful self, the agentic patient who plays with the intubating tube, alongside the self who is in chains that 'pin' and 'bind' and for whom 'sometimes it's too much'. There is ambiguity in the raucous laughter and tears—a reminder of how humour often results from heightened emotions and incongruity. Or we may hear inner contradictions; the 'absent but implicit'[29] of the word 'peace', with its undercur-rent of turbulence. I hear my own voices; my voice of 'hope' with its implications of uncertainty and fear. I hear Pat as she speaks, 'I want to be alive'; I note her use of the present tense, and ponder the meanings of 'alive'. I hear the echoes of the voices of those who said to me, 'Well at least you're alive' and my internal response to that. If we listen carefully, we can hear the whisper of, 'Well, actually, there were times when I wished I had died'. As Bakhtin[30] writes, 'Our practical everyday speech is full of other people's words: with some of them, we completely merge our own voice' (p. 195).

The intersubjective nature of reality is such that meanings are continually shifting, continually negotiated, in the moment and within the context of a particular set of relationships. If we look again at Pat's story, we can see how it is socially and culturally informed and located: the story implicitly embodies the discourse of popular culture; for example, when Pat uses the phrase the 'idea image'[31] (p. 91) of 'biker blokes' and the cultural reference to the band ZZ Top, I immediately have some sense of what I assume to be the picture she intends to convey, an image that is 'out there' in contemporary Western culture. Another instance is the 'idea image' of the 'girl' on her Harley Davidson; these all draw on a particular cultural repertoire. Pat's story also includes medical discourse in, for example, her reference to the 50:50 chance, the quantifying of medical risk, and her sense that such quantifying of risk would have meaning for someone of a certain age within a certain culture.

DIFFERENCES BETWEEN COUNSELLING AND RESEARCH

Since Yasmin was seeing her counsellor at the time of participating in this research, I was curious to find out how these compared and asked her if she experienced differences between counselling and research conversations. She observed:

> I think the biggest difference is that I'm telling you this story ... and I know that you're gonna write it down ... so it's almost like I can remove myself from it. And if I was with my counsellor, that's a chance to talk about things that are a problem at that time. This is more like I'm telling the story, and I'm going back over the last fifteen years. Like the intensive care thing—when I lived through that, it was awful—it was the worst ever time of my life, but I suppose it's over. I've done it. I've got through it and I'm still here. But it's the same, in that with Claire from the first moment I felt I could say anything, and I have that with you as well. I haven't discussed how I felt in any detail with anyone, but with you and with Claire, I feel I can tell you without being judged.
>
> Last time we met—I thought about things we said, and when I got this transcript, I read it and it was almost therapeutic to actually talk about it and to read it. And when I read it I thought to myself, "It's no wonder I'm like I am today; my god I've been through so much". And to see it written down makes me realise that underneath it all I must be a very strong person really. So this has been very beneficial. It's pretty amazing really to see it all together rather than just seeing one episode at a time ...'

When I asked her if she could feel a sense of pride in this, she replied:

> Definitely ... and I really believe that there's not many people could have all this happen to them ... and ... I know I don't have much of a life but I still get up every morning. I still do get through every day, and maybe it's a struggle ... and it is. But I still do it.

REFLECTIONS THAT MAY BE OF USE TO COUNSELLORS MOVING FROM THERAPEUTIC TO RESEARCH CONVERSATIONS

Yasmin's observations above will, I am sure, be of great relevance to both counsellors and researchers. As a counsellor moving into research, I will reflect further on the challenges I have encountered. My assumptions about what constitutes a therapeutic relationship have certainly been challenged; as Yasmin observes, the research relationship can be both validating of a person's experience and can enhance awareness of personal resources. I have realised how valuable it is for someone to read their own story, if it is—as I hope and intend—represented in a way that is as respectful and close to her/his experience as s/he knows it.

In developing the skills and the qualities that I have needed to undertake this narrative inquiry, I have undoubtedly changed as a counsellor. As well as learning to use questions and to draw on my own resonance in ways that I would not have done previously, I have become more aware of the implicit assumptions of my core theoretical model, the person-centred approach. I have had to think about and articulate my taken-for-granted ontological and epistemological assumptions, and to reconcile them with contemporary critical thinking. While I had intuitively felt such reconciliation was possible, I would have neither been aware of, nor able to articulate, the tension I felt between my views of selfhood and spirituality, and the ideas of social constructionism and post-structuralism.

The challenges faced by a counsellor moving from therapeutic to research conversations will vary according to core theoretical model, but will also be influenced by other factors such as personal style. I would certainly suggest that counsellors moving into research could expect personal changes and also changes within their counselling practice. I am aware that as a counsellor, I would work differently, and I regard this as entirely consistent with the person-centred approach. While it was developed by Rogers primarily during the 1960s and 1970s and was contextualised within the values and ideologies of that period, it also incorporates values and thinking that are consistent with more pluralist and postmodern epistemologies. If I am congruent, accepting and empathic as a counsellor, then those qualities include an awareness of sociocultural influences and of issues of knowledge and power.

DIALOGUE BETWEEN THE TEXT AND READER

I have emphasised the relational dimension of this research throughout this book, and just as I believe it has been crucial to be fully present as people have told me their stories, so it has been important to be equally 'present', and to stay close to the spirits of the storytellers in my representations of their stories. Plummer[32] (p. 196) suggests that 'the human sciences should face the daunting task of learning how to communicate in more popular and accessible ways'. I have been aware throughout this study of the tensions, difficulties and ethical dilemmas involved in representing the complexity and continuing nature of individual experience as a finished product. In Chapter Ten I described a performative dimension in my representation of participants' stories. Stories are performative in the sense that we tell them to others in order to initiate or call for responses. As Leach[33] writes, 'It is the connection, the shared exchange that activates the story: interactivity that creates meaning that is more than the self' (p. 19). Jackson Browne[34] has said he knows a 'song is working if people think it's about them … if the song is really doing its job then they're not imagining you in the song, they're imagining themselves in it'. Each one of us will read or hear stories differently, through the filter of our own consciousness, our particular frame of reference, our ways of construing the world. Jane Speedy, at the University of Bristol, frequently, and to great effect, cites Clarissa Pinkola Estes:[35]

> Among my people, questions are often answered with stories. The first story almost always evokes another, which summons another, until the answer to the question has become several stories long. A sequence of tales is thought to offer broader and deeper insight than a single story alone. (p. i)

After presenting Jan's story of the relationship between her illness experience and her professional identity as a psychologist at conferences, I asked if anyone had any questions or responses. Several people responded with their own stories. Some 'witnessed' Jan's story from the position of patient, others from the perspective of healthcare practitioner. A psychologist told a very touching professional identity story of her own, and talked of her awareness of 'pulling rank' and of how 'the story gave me goose bumps … I feel terrible, but I think I've used my status'.

As these responses suggest, while the knowledge gained through stories is, as McCormack[36] notes, 'situated, transient, partial and provisional' (p. 220), the meaning can extend beyond the personal or local context. Stories, as Etherington[37] notes, can 'resonate with others and outlast their telling or reading, and sometimes have profound consequences. They change us in ways we may not always anticipate because they can move us emotionally, change public and political attitudes and opinions, and sometimes influence future actions'.

Bakhtin,[38] in words reminiscent of Buber's *I-It* relationship, describes Devushkin, a character in one of Dostoevsky's stories who was 'outraged that he had been *spied upon* [original emphasis] that his entire life had been analyzed and described, that he had been defined once and for all, that he had been left with no other prospects' (p. 58).

As I have worked with participants' stories and tried to find means of representation that does justice to experience, while at the same time speaking to academic or professional audiences, as I have negotiated the intersubjectivities and the tensions between voices, representation and audience, I have tried to remain aware that when we presume to research people's lives, that when we analyse and describe, we risk defining and thereby reducing and limiting. Frank's[39] concept of 'thinking with' stories seems to me to be close to the dialogic 'way of being' advocated by Rogers and Buber; this involves a genuine interest in and engagement with others that embodies acceptance and empathy alongside an openness and willingness to respond, as researchers, as healthcare practitioners, as readers of a text and above all as fellow human beings.

PERSONAL REFLECTION

In the last 15 years, and through the course of this research, I have been fortunate to have been able to discover and develop new ways of being I could never have envisaged when I was first diagnosed in 1993. Like Church[40] (p. 129), 'The act of writing my illness has been transformative … I write these words from inside a different relationship to my body than I had when I wrote my initial illness' story'. I have travelled a long way from the uncertain beginnings of my research journey, and gained confidence in myself as a social and academic being. I have explored territory of which I had "fleeting awareness" but whose nature was "largely unknown"[41] (p. 13). To paraphrase Eliot,[42] I have arrived back where I started and am coming to know the place, if not for the first time, then certainly with a richer understanding of what it is to be in the position of patient. I have been profoundly moved by the stories told by my participants. I feel my understanding of the uniqueness and complexity of serious illness has been enriched not only by hearing these stories, but also by working to develop a means of representation that conveyed, as closely as possible, a sense of each person. In working to bring experience to life on the page, I am also convinced of both the unique as well as the socially embedded nature of our conceptions of self. Illness illuminates the indivisibility of our intentionality and agency from the cultural and institutional contexts we inhabit. It underlines the contingency of being human, and the relevance of taking into account issues of power and knowledge, which lie at the heart of systems of healthcare.

We are all subject to the contingencies of our fragile bodies, as well as to pervasive and powerful cultural norms. Our bodies, as Oakley[43] writes, are 'both material objects and the site of human experience … It takes accidents, illness, ageing, child-bearing or some other disruption of our normal unconsciousness of the body to make us aware of our bodily integrity' (pp. 15–16). Illness reminds us of the universality of our contingent embodiment; becoming patients underlines the social implications of that embodiment.

The song that crystallises the infinity of meanings, intuitions and synchronicities suspended within the 'spider web' and 'silk threads'[44] (p. 2) of my own consciousness—my 'Desert Island disc' for all time—is *Sky Blue and Black* by Jackson Browne.[45] It was in my head and in my heart throughout the time I was in hospital for my surgery in February 1994. There is a heart-breaking sadness in his voice, in the melody and in the poignancy of the recurring phrase he plays on the piano. The words capture my feeling of the utter contingency of life, and of how illness can send us in directions we could not have anticipated, and from which there is no going back. Such contingency has opened up new possibilities for living that would have been unimaginable to me 15 years ago. I have been given a precious opportunity to live a meaningful and rewarding life, and I am deeply grateful for that, and for the privilege of working with Pat, Jan, Jim and Yasmin.

REFERENCES

1. Bruner J. *Actual Minds, Possible Worlds*. Cambridge, MA: Harvard University Press; 1986.
2. Spiro HM, McCrea C, Curnen MG, *et al.*, editors. *Empathy and the Practice of Medicine*. London: Yale University Press; 1993.
3. Levinas E. *Outside the Subject*. London: The Athlone Press; 1993.
4. Bruner J. *Making Stories: law, literature, life*. New York: Farrar, Straus and Giroux; 2002. p. 70–2.
5. White M. Re-engaging with history: the absent but implicit. In: White M, editor. *Reflections on Narrative Practice: essays and interviews*. Adelaide: Dulwich Centre Publications; 2000.
6. White M and Epston D *Narrative Means to Therapeutic Ends*. New York: Norton; 1990.
7. Etherington K. *Narrative Approaches to Working with Male Survivors of Sexual Abuse: the clients', the counsellor's and the researcher's story*. London: Jessica Kingsley; 2000.
8. Etherington K. Working together: editing a book as narrative research methodology. *Counsell Psychother Res J*. 2002b; 2(3).
9. Etherington K. *Trauma, the Body and Transformation*. London: Jessica Kingsley; 2003.
10. Etherington K. *Becoming a Reflexive Researcher: using our selves in research*. London: Jessica Kingsley; 2004.
11. Etherington K. *Trauma, Drug Misuse and Transforming Identities*. London: Jessica Kingsley; 2008.
12. Payne M. *Narrative Therapy: an introduction for counsellors*. London: Sage; 2002.
13. Speedy J. The storied helper: an introduction to narrative ideas in counselling and psychotherapy. *Eur J Psychother Counsell Health*. 2000; 3(3): 361–75.
14. Speedy J. *Narrative Inquiry and Psychotherapy*. Basingstoke: Palgrave Macmillan; 2008.
15. Anderson H, Goolishian H. The client is the expert: a not-knowing approach to therapy. In: McNamee S, Gergen K, editors. *Therapy as Social Construction*. London: Sage; 1992. pp. 25–39.
16. Gergen K. Therapeutic professions and the diffusion of deficit. *J Mind Behav*. 1990; 11: 353–68.
17. Martin V. Dialogue in the narrative process. *J Med Ethics*. 33: 49–54.
18. Foucault M. Of other spaces. *Diacritics*. 1986 Spring; 16: 22–7.
19. Buber M. *I and Thou*. Edinburgh: T&T Clark; 1937.
20. Kirschenbaum H, Henderson V, editors. *The Carl Rogers Reader*. London: Constable; 1990.
21. Foucault, op cit.

22. Buber, 1937, op cit.
23. *Between Man and Man.* London: Routledge Classics; 1947.
24. Rogers CR. *A Way of Being.* Boston, MA: Houghton Mifflin; 1980.
25. Frank A. What is dialogical research and why should we do it? *Qual Heal Res.* 2005; 15(7): 964–74.
26. Frank A. *The Wounded Storyteller: body, illness and ethics.* Chicago, IL: University of Chicago Press; 1995.
27. Foucault, op cit.
28. Bakhtin M. *Problems of Dostoevsky's Poetics.* Emerson C, translator, editor. Manchester: Manchester University Press; 1984.
29. White, 2000, op cit.
30. Bakhtin M. *Problems of Dostoevsky's Poetics.* Emerson C, translator, editor. Minneapolis, MN: University of Minnesota Press; 1997.
31. Bakhtin, 1984, op cit.
32. Plummer K. *Documents of Life 2: an invitation to critical humanism.* London: Sage; 2001.
33. Leach H. Crossing the line: stories on mapping the maze. *Times Higher Education Supplement.* 2004 Nov 5. pp. 18–19.
34. Browne J. *Uncut* [recording]. 2002 Dec.
35. Estes, CP. *The Gift of Story.* New York, NY: Rider; 1993.
36. McCormack C. Storying stories: a narrative approach to in-depth interview conversations. *Int J Soc Res Meth.* 2004; 7: 219–36.
37. Etherington K. BASPR [keynote]. 2008.
38. Bakhtin, 1984, op cit.
39. Frank, 1995, op cit.
40. Church, K. *Forbidden Narratives: critical autobiography as social science.* London: Gordon and Breach; 1995.
41. Moustakas C. *Heuristic Research: design, methodology and applications.* Thousand Oaks, CA: Sage; 1990.
42. Eliot TS. *Little Gidding. The Complete Poems and Plays.* London: Faber and Faber; 1969.
43. Oakley A. *Fracture: adventures of a broken body.* Bristol: The Policy Press; 2007.
44. James H. The Art of Fiction. In: *Partial Portraits.* New York, NY: Macmillan; 1888.
45. Browne J. Sky Blue and Black. *I'm Alive* [recording]. Elektra; 1993.

Index